# THE SIMPLE 5-INGREDIENT BARIATRIC COOKBOOK FOR BEGINNERS

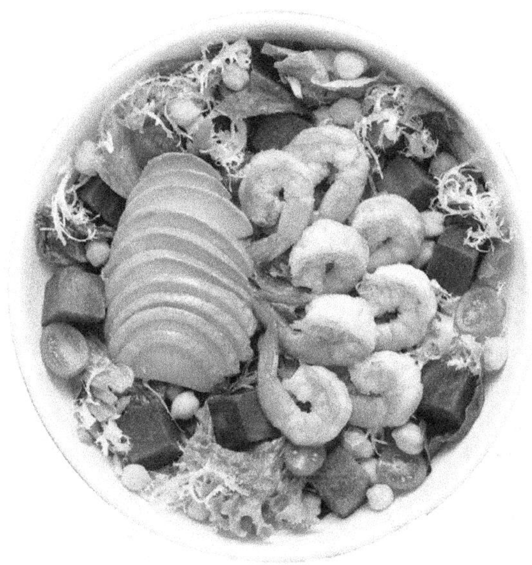

*Fast, Healthy, and Simple 5-Ingredient Meals to Support Your Weight Loss Journey After Gastric Sleeve Surgery with Everyday Supermarket Items*

**Joan G. Milone**

## Copyright © 2024 by Joan G. Milone

## All rights reserved.

This book is written as a source of information only. The information contained in this book is provided in good faith and is believed to be accurate and reliable as of the date of publication. The author does not assume any responsibility for any errors or omissions that may appear.

## SCAN TO ACCESS MORE AMAZING COOKBOOKS FROM JOAN

# Table of Contents

## Dinner — 41



## Snacks and Sides — 51



## Desserts — 59



## Meat and Poultry — 69

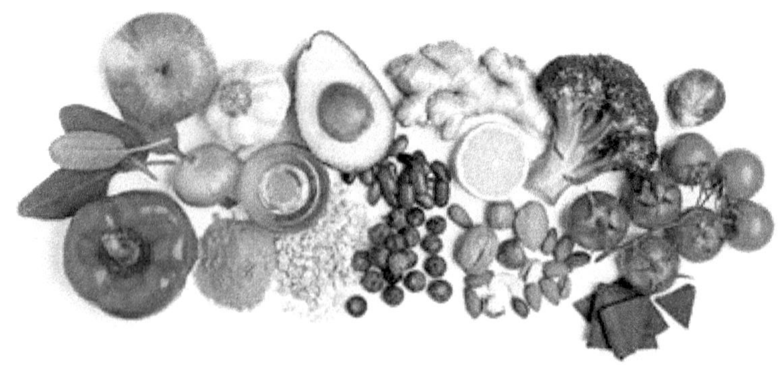

# Introduction

Welcome to "The Simple 5-Ingredient Bariatric Cookbook for Beginners," a tasty, simple, and healthy culinary adventure developed specifically for you. Whether you're new to post-gastric sleeve surgery or simply searching for a healthier, more manageable approach to your meals, this book is your guide.

Imagine standing in front of your cabinet or refrigerator, unsure what to prepare, anxious about nutritional balance, portion sizes, and, most importantly, the intricacy of dishes to meet your new dietary requirements. It is a struggle that many people experience, but I am here to tell you that it does not have to be overwhelming. Consider this book to be a helpful guide, taking you by the hand and reassuring you that with only five basic ingredients, you can make meals that not only support your health journey but also satisfy your taste buds.

Let me share a story that inspired me to create this cookbook. A close friend underwent gastric sleeve surgery and faced overwhelming confusion about what to eat during recovery. Watching their struggle, I realized there was a dire need for a simple, straightforward guide to eating well after bariatric surgery. This realization was the spark that ignited my passion for crafting this book. I dove into research, consulted with dietitians specializing in post-bariatric nutrition, and experimented in my own kitchen to bring these recipes to life.

This cookbook is more than just a collection of recipes; it's a companion on your journey to a healthier you. Our adventure will begin with breakfast, the most essential meal of the day, laying the groundwork for a satisfying and invigorating start. We'll look at lunches that are ideal for on-the-go, dinners that provide comfort at the end of a hard day, and snacks and sides that alleviate those hunger pains in between meals. And, because life is about balance, we'll indulge in sweets that satisfy your sweet craving while staying on track with your health objectives. Along the way, we'll cover meats, poultry, soups, salads, fish, shellfish, and even drinks, with each part including dishes created with only five simple ingredients.

Beyond recipes, this book provides advice on portion control, nutritional consumption, and navigating store aisles to make the best choices. You'll discover meal planning and preparation techniques to help you streamline your weekly eating routine.

So, to you, the reader, who may be feeling a little confused in the kitchen after surgery or simply looking for an easier method to eat healthy, let's go on this culinary journey together. My objective is for you to rediscover the joy of cooking and eating, and to feel empowered and thrilled about the possibilities that simplicity offers. Here's to a voyage of knowledge, health, and, most importantly, great meals that will make you smile. Welcome aboard!

## Understanding the Gastric Sleeve Diet: Phases and Principles

Understanding the diet following gastric sleeve surgery is critical for a full recovery and long-term weight maintenance. The gastric sleeve diet is painstakingly planned to assist your body to recuperate correctly while adjusting to your new stomach capacity. It is separated into various phases, each with its own set of principles and goals, to ensure that you obtain all of the nutrients you need without overwhelming your newly altered digestive system.

**Phases of the Gastric Sleeve Diet.**

**1. Liquid Phase (1-2 weeks post-surgery):** The initial phase involves drinking clear, sugar-free liquids to stay hydrated and promote healing. Clear liquids, broth, and unsweetened tea are all options. This phase allows your stomach to begin the mending process without being stretched by solid meals.

**2. Pureed Foods Phase (weeks 3-4):** As your body adjusts, switch to pureed foods that are smooth and free of solid parts to reduce stomach strain. Pureed fruits and vegetables, as well as lean proteins, are provided to ensure that you obtain the vitamins and nutrients your body requires for recuperation.

**3. Soft meals Phase (weeks 5-8):** Easy-to-digest soft meals are the next step. This includes soft fruits, veggies, and tender meats. The idea is to gradually reintroduce solid meals into your digestive system while avoiding any hard, crunchy, or fibrous foods that may disturb the healing process.

**4. Solid meals Phase:** After successfully completing the preceding phases, progressively incorporate more solid meals into your diet. This phase emphasizes nutrient-dense foods to maintain a balanced diet, particularly lean meats, fruits, vegetables, and whole grains. Portion management is critical because your stomach's capacity has considerably decreased.

**Principles of the Gastric Sleeve Diet**

- **Nutrient Density:** Prioritize foods rich in nutrients to meet your body's needs with smaller portions. Protein is particularly important for healing and muscle maintenance.

- **Hydration:** Drinking enough fluids is crucial, but avoid drinking 30 minutes before or after meals to avoid expanding your stomach and diluting digestive enzymes.

- **Mindful Eating:** Eat slowly, chew carefully, and identify when you're full to prevent overeating and putting strain on your stomach.

- **Supplementation:** Vitamin and mineral supplements are frequently required to prevent nutritional deficits caused by decreased food intake and absorption.

- **Avoiding Empty Calories:** Limit your consumption of foods heavy in sugar and fat that have little nutritional value, since they can impede weight reduction and recovery.

Understanding and following the phases and concepts of the gastric sleeve diet is critical for a successful recovery and attaining your long-term health and weight control objectives. This systematic method reduces difficulties, promotes sustainable eating habits, and opens the road to a healthy lifestyle following surgery.

## Tips for Post-Bariatric Surgery Nutrition

Certainly, a post-bariatric surgery diet is an important part of your weight reduction journey and general health. Here are some important guidelines to help you maintain a healthy and balanced diet following surgery:

1. **Follow Your Surgeon's Recommendations:** Always follow the dietary restrictions prescribed by your surgeon or healthcare team. These rules are particular to your operation and requirements.

2. **Begin Slowly:** After surgery, your stomach will be smaller, and your digestive system may require time to adjust. Start with clear liquids, then graduate to full liquids, and then to soft and solid meals as directed.

3. **Portion Management:** Even with a smaller stomach, it is critical to exercise portion management. Avoid overeating since it might cause discomfort and difficulties.

4. **Protein Priority:** Eat protein-rich meals including lean meats, fish, poultry, tofu, and lentils. Protein aids in the recovery and maintenance of muscle mass.

5. **Limit Sugar and High-Fat meals:** Sugary and high-fat meals might cause weight gain and digestive problems. Reduce or eliminate them from your diet.

6. **Stay Hydrated:** Drink lots of water throughout the day to maintain hydration. Dehydration can cause difficulties and prevent weight loss.

7. **Chew Fully:** Chewing your meal fully is vital for digestion and avoiding discomfort. Take your time during mealtimes.

8. **Nutrient-Dense Foods:** Include fruits and vegetables, whole grains, and low-fat dairy. These foods include critical vitamins and minerals.

9. **Supplements:** Depending on your operation, you may need to take vitamin and mineral supplements to avoid deficiencies.

10. **Listen to Your Body.** Pay attention to hunger and fullness cues. Eat just when you are hungry, and quit when you are full.

11. **Regular Follow-Ups:** Make regular consultations with your healthcare team to track your progress and discuss any issues.

12. **Exercise:** Include regular physical exercise in your daily routine, as prescribed by your healthcare professional. Exercise is vital for weight control and general health.

13. **Emotional Help:** Seek emotional help from a counselor or a support group to address any emotional or psychological issues connected to weight loss and body image.

14. **Meal Planning:** Plan your meals and snacks ahead of time to help you make healthy choices and prevent impulsive eating.

15. **Be Patient:** Weight reduction following surgery takes time. Be patient with yourself, keep focused on your goals, and enjoy your accomplishments along the road.

Remember that a post-bariatric surgery diet requires a lifetime commitment to your health and well-being. By following these guidelines and collaborating with your healthcare team, you may reach and sustain your weight reduction goals while living a healthier and more happy life.

## The Benefits of a 5-Ingredient Approach

Adopting a 5-ingredient post-gastric sleeve surgery diet has several advantages, both for your physical health and your general lifestyle.

This strategy simplifies meal planning and preparation, allowing you to stay on track with your nutritional requirements while also making your meals pleasurable and rewarding. Here are some of the main benefits of following this minimalist cooking philosophy:

**Simpler Meal Preparation**

**Ease of Cooking:** Recipes with only five ingredients are fundamentally easier, requiring less time and effort to make meals. This simplicity is especially useful when you're transitioning to a new eating style and searching for methods to make healthy eating more accessible and time-efficient.

**Reduced Grocery Shopping Stress:** Buying fewer ingredients makes your excursions to the grocery more manageable. It allows you to focus on buying high-quality, nutritious meals without being distracted by long and convoluted ingredient lists.

**Enhanced Nutritional Focus**

**Quality Over Quantity:** Limiting the number of ingredients encourages the selection of nutrient-dense foods, ensuring that each component of your meal has a function in your diet. This is especially essential following gastric sleeve surgery, as optimizing nutrition in lower meal sizes is critical.

**Easier Portion Regulate:** Smaller ingredient lists typically result in simpler meals, making it easier to regulate portion amounts and follow dietary requirements after surgery. This can help with weight control and lower the chance of overeating.

## Psychological and Emotional Benefits.

**Reduced Decision Fatigue:** Using fewer ingredients and simpler dishes reduces the burden of selecting what to eat. This may make meals more fun and less like a chore, promoting a better relationship with food.

**Creativity and Experimentation:** With only five ingredients, you must think imaginatively about how to utilize them in different ways, resulting in a fun and experimental approach to cooking. This may reignite your passion for food and cooking, making meals something to look forward to.

## Financial Savings

**Cost-Effective:** Buying fewer ingredients for each meal can lead to significant savings over time. This approach encourages the use of whole, unprocessed foods, which are often more economical than their processed counterparts.

## Supports Long-Term Health Goals.

**Consistent Healthy Eating:** The 5-ingredient method's simplicity makes it simpler to keep to a healthy eating plan, promoting long-term weight control and nutritional goals. It promotes a sustainable approach to eating properly, which is critical following bariatric surgery.

In essence, a 5-ingredient strategy meets the demands of those who have had gastric sleeve surgery. It provides a practical, fun, and long-term approach to meeting nutritional objectives, streamlining the cooking process, and maintaining a happy and healthy connection with food.

## How to Use This Cookbook

Using "The Simple 5-Ingredient Bariatric Cookbook for Beginners" is intended to be simple and powerful, allowing you to manage your post-surgery diet with confidence. Here's how you get the most out of this cookbook in five simple steps:

**1. Understand the Introduction.**

Begin by reading the introduction to learn about the theory behind the 5-ingredient method, the cookbook's layout, and how it is suited to your specific needs following gastric sleeve surgery.

**2. Explore the Phases and Principles.**

Before getting into the recipes, acquaint yourself with the dietary stages following gastric sleeve surgery and the nutritional guidelines stated in the book. This knowledge will assist you in selecting recipes suited for your current state of rehabilitation and ensuring that your meals promote your health and recuperation.

## 3. Plan Your Meals.

Use the cookbook to plan your weekly meals. Begin by picking dishes from the relevant areas for your current dietary phase. Include a variety of meals to maintain a healthy diet and keep mealtime interesting. The recipes are simple enough that you may plan and prepare your meals ahead of time, which will help you remain on track.

## 4. Cook with Confidence.

Each dish is basic and clear, with step-by-step directions that make cooking accessible to everyone, including beginners. Don't be scared to experiment with the recipes and make changes based on your tastes and nutritional requirements. The idea is to gain confidence in the kitchen while eating tasty, nutritious meals.

## 5. Reflect and Adjust.

After sampling a meal, take a minute to consider how it fits into your diet, how it makes you feel, and any changes you might want to make next time. Your preferences and tolerances may vary as you continue through your post-surgery recovery, and this cookbook is intended to evolve with you. Use it to learn about your new dietary requirements, find new favorite meals, and enjoy the process of preparing and eating healthily.

Following these steps will transform "The Simple 5-Ingredient Bariatric Cookbook for Beginners" into more than simply a collection of recipes; it will serve as a guide on your journey to a healthier, more enjoyable way of eating after gastric sleeve surgery.

## Cooking Techniques and Kitchen Tools

Here are some essential techniques and tools to consider:

**Cooking Techniques:**

**1. Grilling:** Grilling is a healthy cooking method that adds flavor without excess fat. Grill lean proteins like chicken, fish, and vegetables for a delicious meal.

**2. Baking:** Baking is a versatile method that can be used for proteins, vegetables, and healthy desserts. Use a non-stick baking sheet or silicone mat to reduce the need for added fats.

**3. Steaming:** Steaming is a gentle cooking method that preserves nutrients in vegetables and proteins. Invest in a steamer basket or use a microwave-safe steaming container.

**4. Sautéing:** Sautéing with a small amount of oil or cooking spray is a quick way to cook vegetables and proteins. A non-stick skillet is handy for this technique.

**5. Roasting:** Roasting vegetables enhances their flavor. Use a roasting pan or a baking sheet with raised edges to prevent juices from spilling.

**6. Blending:** Blenders are great for making smoothies, soups, and sauces. Invest in a high-quality blender for smooth and consistent results.

**7. Food Processor:** A food processor can simplify meal prep by chopping, slicing, and dicing ingredients quickly.

**8. Slow Cooking:** A slow cooker allows you to prepare meals with minimal effort. It's perfect for soups, stews, and tenderizing tougher cuts of meat.

**Kitchen Tools:**

**1. Kitchen Scale:** A digital kitchen scale helps you accurately measure portion sizes and ingredients.

**2. Measuring Cups and Spoons:** These are essential for precise measurements when cooking and baking.

**3. Non-Stick Cookware:** Non-stick pans and baking sheets reduce the need for excess oil and make cooking and cleanup easier.

**4. Steamer Basket:** If you steam vegetables frequently, a steamer basket is a useful tool.

**5. Chef's Knife:** A good-quality chef's knife makes chopping and slicing easier and safer.

**6. Cutting Boards:** Invest in cutting boards made of materials like wood or plastic for food safety and easy cleaning.

**7. Vegetable Peeler:** A vegetable peeler is handy for peeling and slicing vegetables and fruits.

**8. Food Thermometer:** Ensure your proteins are cooked safely by using a food thermometer to check internal temperatures.

**9. Blender or Food Processor:** Choose one or both based on your cooking needs.

**10. Slow Cooker:** For convenient meal preparation.

**11. Mixing Bowls:** A set of mixing bowls in various sizes is versatile for food prep.

**12. Tongs:** Tongs are useful for flipping and handling food in hot pans.

**13. Colander:** Use a colander for draining pasta, rinsing vegetables, and more.

**14. Silicone Utensils:** Non-scratch silicone utensils are safe to use with non-stick cookware.

**15. Storage Containers:** Invest in a variety of airtight storage containers for storing prepped ingredients and leftovers.

**16. Can Opener:** If you use canned ingredients, a reliable can opener is essential.

**17. Microwave-Safe Dishes:** These are handy for reheating and steaming in the microwave.

**18. Oven Mitts and Pot Holders:** Ensure safety when handling hot cookware.

By mastering these cooking techniques and having the right kitchen tools, you'll be well-equipped to prepare delicious, healthy meals that align with your bariatric dietary guidelines. Experiment with different cooking methods and find what works best for your tastes and lifestyle.

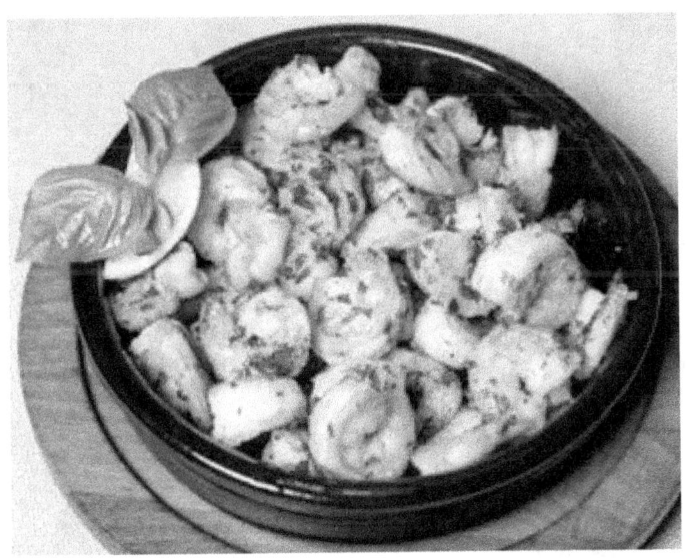

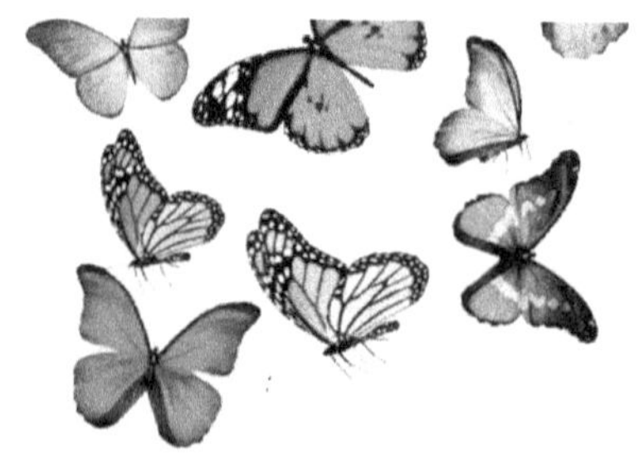

"Every bite is a step towards your new beginning. Embrace the journey with joy and patience. Your health is worth every effort."

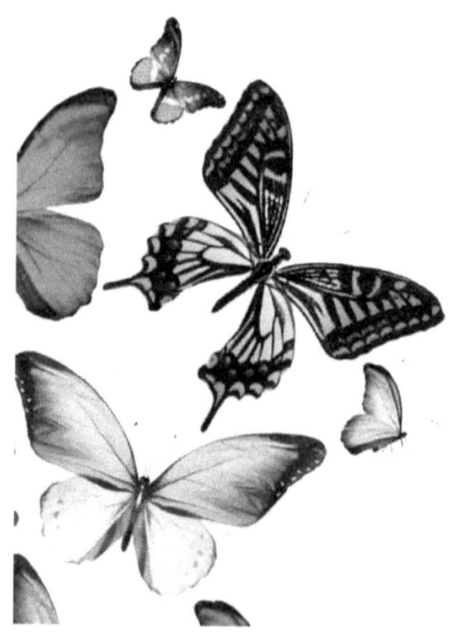

# Breakfast

**B**reakfast is frequently cited as the most crucial meal of the day, and this is especially true after gastric sleeve surgery. This section is intended to start your day with nutritious, easy-to-prepare meals that meet your new dietary restrictions. Each dish is carefully prepared with only five ingredients, assuring simplicity without losing flavor or nutritional value. These breakfast alternatives are not only bariatric-friendly, but also delicious and diverse, ensuring that your mornings are both fun and nutritious. Let's go on a journey to make breakfast a satisfying and invigorating start to your day every day.

## Protein-Packed Greek Yogurt Parfait

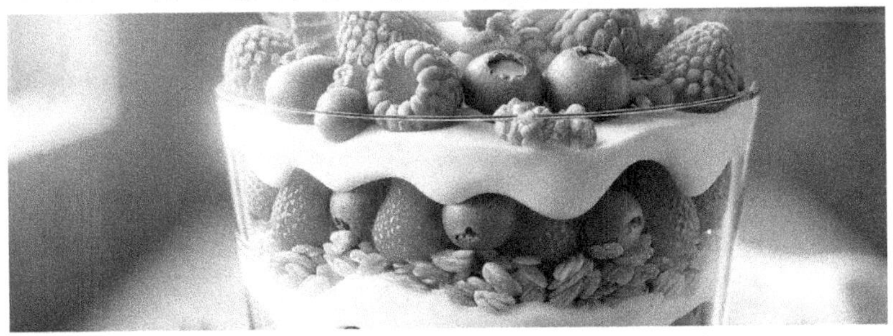

## Ingredients:

- 1 cup plain Greek yogurt (low-fat)
- ½ cup mixed berries (strawberries, blueberries, raspberries)
- 2 tablespoons granola (low-sugar)
- 1 tablespoon honey
- 1 teaspoon chia seeds

## Preparation:

1. In a serving glass, layer half of the Greek yogurt at the bottom.
2. Add a layer of mixed berries over the yogurt.
3. Sprinkle 1 tablespoon of granola and half of the chia seeds.
4. Repeat the layers with the remaining yogurt, berries, granola, and chia seeds.
5. Drizzle honey over the top for added sweetness.

**Cooking Time:** No cooking required; preparation time is about 5 minutes.

**Nutritional Values** (approximate per serving):

- Calories: 250
- Protein: 20g
- Carbohydrates: 35g
- Fat: 5g
- Fiber: 4g
- Sugar: 25g (check labels to adjust for added sugars in yogurt and granola)

**Rating: ★★★★★**

This parfait combines the richness of Greek yogurt with the freshness of berries and the crunch of granola, offering a balanced and nutritious start to your day. It's perfect for a quick breakfast or a refreshing snack, providing a good balance of protein, healthy fats, and carbohydrates.

## Savory Spinach and Feta Egg Muffins

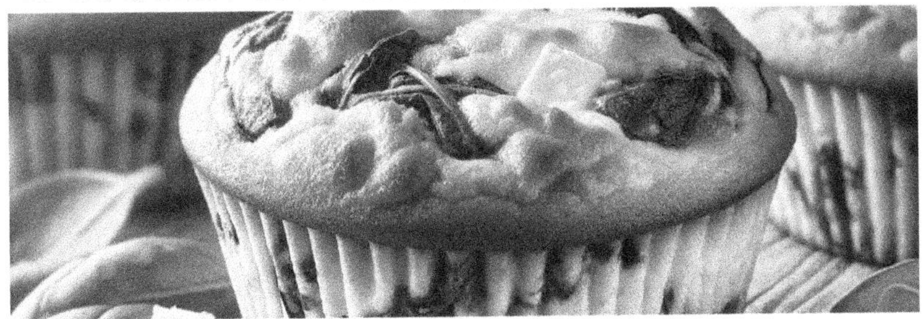

**Ingredients:**

- 6 large eggs
- 1 cup fresh spinach, chopped
- 1/2 cup feta cheese, crumbled
- Salt and pepper to taste
- Non-stick cooking spray

**Preparation:**

1. Preheat the oven to 350°F (175°C) and prepare a muffin tin by spraying it with non-stick cooking spray.
2. In a large bowl, whisk the eggs. Add the chopped spinach and crumbled feta cheese. Season with salt and pepper.

3. Pour the egg mixture evenly into the muffin tin, filling each cup about 3/4 full.

4. Bake in the preheated oven for 20-25 minutes, or until the egg muffins are set and lightly golden on top.

**Cooking Time:** 25 minutes

**Nutritional Values** (approximate per muffin):

- Calories: 100
- Protein: 9g
- Carbohydrates: 2g
- Fat: 7g
- Fiber: 0.5g
- Sugar: 1g

**Rating:** ★★★★★

These Savory Spinach and Feta Egg Muffins are a delicious and nutritious breakfast option, perfect for on-the-go mornings. Packed with protein from the eggs and enriched with the flavors of spinach and feta, they offer a satisfying and healthy start to any day.

## Almond Butter Banana Smoothie

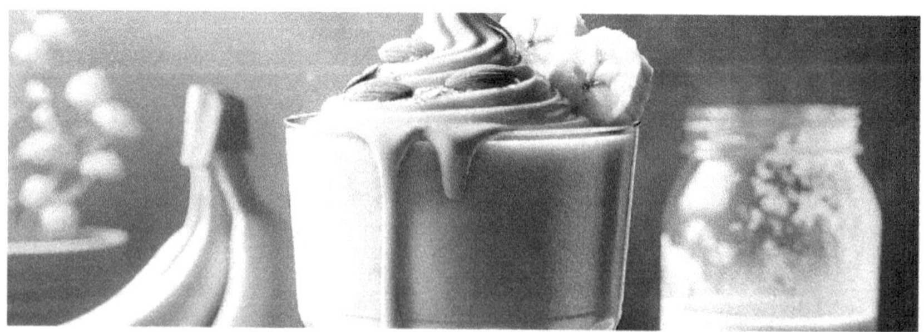

**Ingredients:**

- 1 ripe banana
- 2 tablespoons almond butter
- 1 cup almond milk (unsweetened)
- 1/2 teaspoon vanilla extract
- Ice cubes (optional)

**Preparation:**

1. In a blender, combine the ripe banana, almond butter, unsweetened almond milk, and vanilla extract.
2. Add a handful of ice cubes if you prefer a chilled smoothie.
3. Blend on high until smooth and creamy.

**Cooking Time:** 5 minutes

**Nutritional Values** (approximate per serving):

- Calories: 280
- Protein: 8g
- Carbohydrates: 30g
- Fat: 16g
- Fiber: 5g
- Sugar: 15g

**Rating:** ★★★★★

This Almond Butter Banana Smoothie is a creamy, satisfying blend that makes for a perfect breakfast or snack. Packed with the nutritional benefits of banana and almond butter, it provides a good balance of protein, healthy fats, and natural sweetness. Quick and easy to prepare, it's an ideal option for a nutritious, on-the-go meal.

# Cottage Cheese and Peach Compote

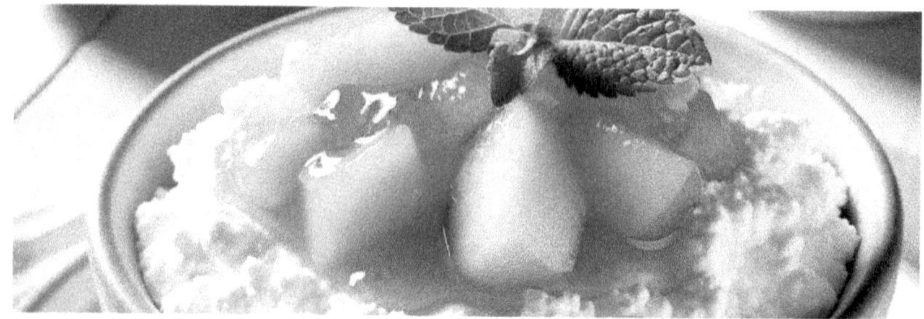

## Ingredients:

- 1 cup cottage cheese (low-fat)
- 1 large peach, sliced
- 1 tablespoon honey
- 1/4 teaspoon cinnamon
- Mint leaves for garnish (optional)

## Preparation:

1. In a small saucepan, combine the peach slices, honey, and cinnamon. Cook over medium heat for 5-7 minutes, or until the peaches are soft and the mixture has thickened slightly.

2. Place the cottage cheese in a serving bowl.

3. Top the cottage cheese with the warm peach compote.

4. Garnish with mint leaves if desired.

**Cooking Time:** 10 minutes

**Nutritional Values** (approximate per serving):

- Calories: 200
- Protein: 15g

- Carbohydrates: 25g
- Fat: 2g
- Fiber: 2g
- Sugar: 22g

**Rating: ★★★★★**

This Cottage Cheese and Peach Compote combines the creamy texture of cottage cheese with the sweetness of peaches, creating a delightful and nutritious dish. Perfect for breakfast or a light snack, it's a simple yet flavorful way to start your day, offering a good balance of protein, vitamins, and a hint of sweetness.

## Avocado Toast with Poached Egg

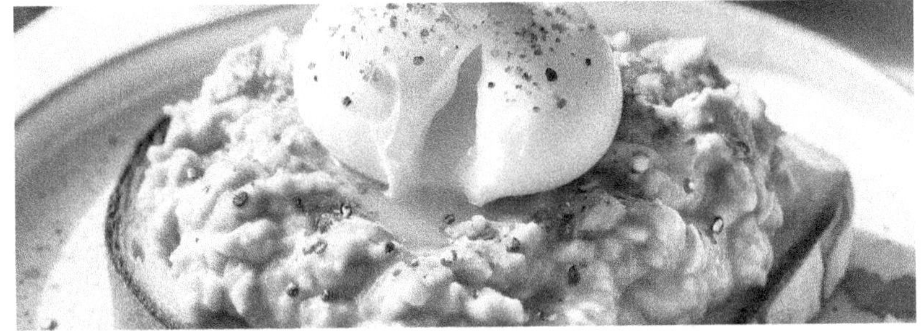

**Ingredients:**

- 1 slice whole grain bread
- 1/2 ripe avocado
- 1 egg
- Salt and pepper to taste
- Chili flakes (optional)

**Preparation:**

1. Toast the whole grain bread to your preference.
2. Mash the avocado and spread it evenly on the toasted bread.

3. Poach the egg by bringing a pot of water to a simmer, gently cracking the egg into the water, and cooking for 3-4 minutes for a runny yolk or longer for a firmer yolk.
4. Place the poached egg on top of the avocado toast.
5. Season with salt, pepper, and chili flakes if desired.

**Cooking Time:** 10 minutes

**Nutritional Values** (approximate per serving):

- Calories: 300
- Protein: 12g
- Carbohydrates: 20g
- Fat: 20g
- Fiber: 7g
- Sugar: 3g

**Rating:** ★★★★★

Avocado Toast with Poached Egg is a modern breakfast classic, offering a perfect blend of heart-healthy fats, high-quality protein, and essential nutrients. This simple yet satisfying meal is not only delicious but also packs a nutritional punch, making it an ideal way to start your day. The combination of creamy avocado, crunchy toast, and a perfectly poached egg is sure to please.

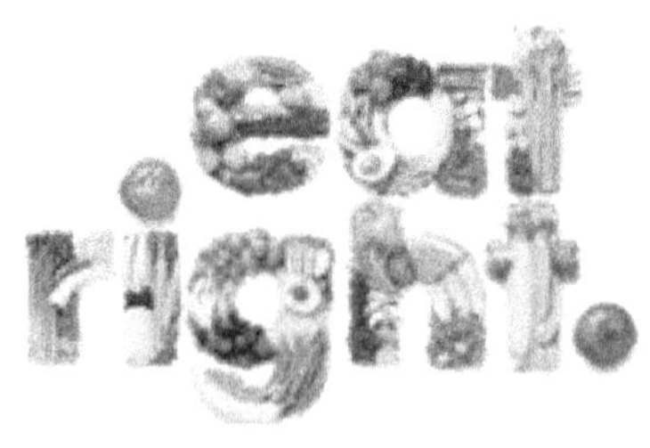

# Lunch

Lunch is a pivotal meal that bridges your morning and evening, providing you with the energy and nutrients needed to power through the day. Our section on lunch recipes is designed with your health and busy schedule in mind. Each dish, crafted with no more than five ingredients, promises a delightful balance of flavor and nutrition, ensuring that you can enjoy a satisfying meal without spending hours in the kitchen. These lunch options cater to your post-gastric sleeve dietary needs, offering a variety of tastes and textures to keep your midday meals interesting and nourishing. Embrace these simple yet delicious recipes to make every lunchtime a moment to look forward to, fueling your body and pleasing your palate.

## Turkey and Avocado Roll-Ups

**Ingredients:**

- 4 slices turkey breast (deli-style, low sodium)
- 1 ripe avocado, sliced
- 1/2 cup spinach leaves

- 1 tablespoon mustard
- Salt and pepper to taste

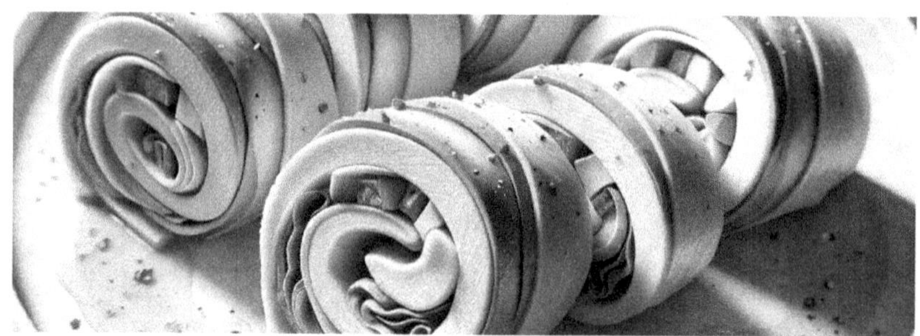

## Preparation:

1. Lay out the turkey slices on a flat surface.

2. Spread a thin layer of mustard on each slice.

3. Place a few avocado slices and spinach leaves on one end of each turkey slice.

4. Season with salt and pepper.

5. Carefully roll up the turkey slices, securing the filling inside.

**Cooking Time:** No cooking required; preparation time is about 10 minutes.

**Nutritional Values** (approximate per serving of 2 roll-ups):

- Calories: 150
- Fat: 9g
- Protein: 12g
- Fiber: 4g
- Carbohydrates: 8g
- Sugar: 1g

**Rating:** ★★★★★

Turkey and Avocado Roll-Ups are a quick, nutritious snack or light meal option, combining lean protein from turkey with the healthy fats of avocado. Easy to prepare and packed with flavor, these roll-ups are perfect for a post-workout snack, a light lunch, or a grab-and-go option.

## Broccoli and Cheddar Soup

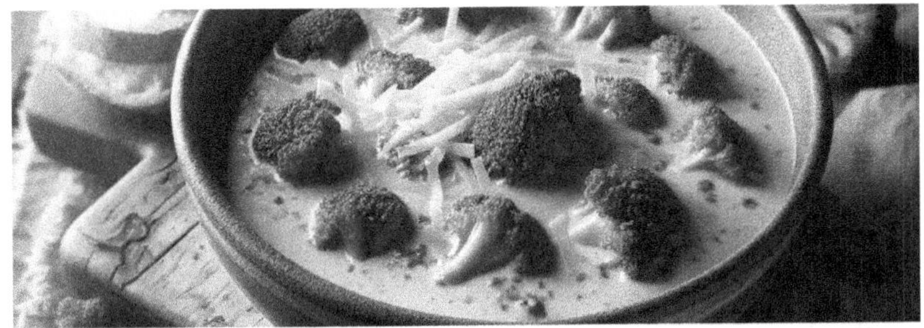

**Ingredients:**

- 2 cups broccoli florets, chopped
- 1 cup chicken or vegetable broth
- 1 cup cheddar cheese, grated
- 1/2 cup heavy cream
- Salt and pepper to taste

**Preparation:**

1. In a medium saucepan, bring the broth to a boil. Add the broccoli florets and simmer until they are tender, about 5-7 minutes.

2. Reduce the heat to low and stir in the heavy cream and grated cheddar cheese until the cheese melts and the soup becomes creamy. Avoid boiling to prevent the cream from curdling.

3. Season with salt and pepper to taste.

4. Use an immersion blender to puree the soup directly in the pot to your desired consistency. Alternatively, carefully transfer to a blender to puree and then return to the pot.

**Cooking Time:** 15 minutes

**Nutritional Values** (approximate per serving):

- Calories: 300
- Protein: 15g
- Carbohydrates: 8g
- Fat: 24g
- Fiber: 2g
- Sugar: 3g

**Rating:** ★★★★★

This Broccoli and Cheddar Soup combines the nutritional benefits of broccoli with the rich, comforting flavors of cheddar cheese and cream. It's a perfect, heartwarming dish for a quick lunch or a soothing dinner, offering a simple yet delicious way to enjoy your veggies.

## Quinoa and Black Bean Salad

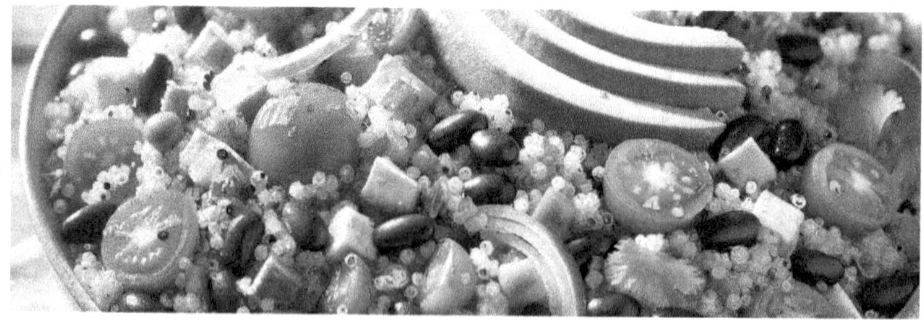

## Ingredients:

- 1 cup cooked quinoa
- 1 cup black beans, rinsed and drained
- 1/2 cup cherry tomatoes, halved
- 2 tablespoons fresh lime juice
- Salt to taste

## Preparation:

1. In a large bowl, combine the cooked quinoa and black beans.
2. Add the halved cherry tomatoes to the bowl.
3. Drizzle with fresh lime juice and gently toss to combine.
4. Season with salt to your liking.

**Cooking Time:** No cooking required if using pre-cooked quinoa; preparation time is about 10 minutes.

**Nutritional Values** (approximate per serving):

- Calories: 220
- Protein: 9g
- Carbohydrates: 40g
- Fat: 2g
- Fiber: 8g
- Sugar: 3g

**Rating: ★★★★★**

This Quinoa and Black Bean Salad, with its simple combination of ingredients, offers a wholesome and flavorful option for a healthy lunch or side dish. The natural sweetness of cherry tomatoes complements the earthiness of black beans and quinoa, while lime juice adds a refreshing zing, making this salad a delightful, nutritious choice.

## Grilled Chicken Caesar Wrap

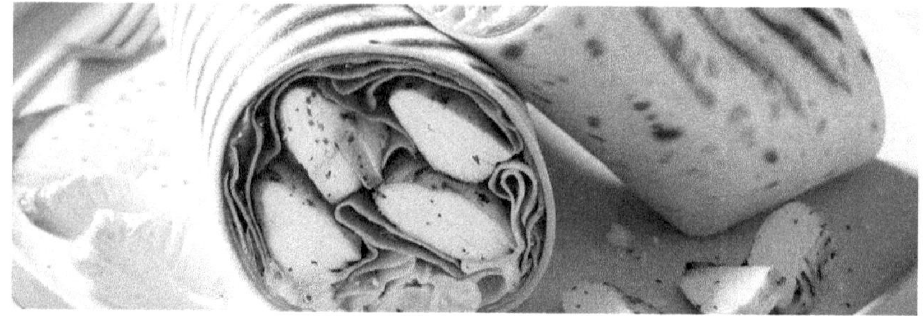

**Ingredients:**

- 1 grilled chicken breast, sliced
- 2 large romaine lettuce leaves
- 2 tablespoons Caesar dressing
- 1/4 cup Parmesan cheese, shaved
- 1 large whole wheat tortilla wrap

**Preparation:**

1. Lay the whole wheat tortilla flat on a plate.
2. Place the romaine lettuce leaves in the center of the tortilla.
3. Add the sliced grilled chicken breast on top of the lettuce.
4. Drizzle the Caesar dressing over the chicken and sprinkle with shaved Parmesan cheese.

5. Carefully fold the tortilla to form a wrap, tucking in the edges to hold the filling.

**Cooking Time:** No cooking required if using pre-grilled chicken; preparation time is about 5 minutes.

**Nutritional Values** (approximate per wrap):

- Calories: 350
- Protein: 30g
- Carbohydrates: 25g
- Fat: 15g
- Fiber: 3g
- Sugar: 2g

**Rating:** ★★★★★

This Grilled Chicken Caesar Wrap combines the classic flavors of a Caesar salad with the convenience of a wrap for a quick and satisfying meal. Perfect for a lunch on the go, it offers a balanced mix of protein, greens, and whole grains, all wrapped up in a delicious, easy-to-eat package.

## Tuna Salad Stuffed Tomatoes

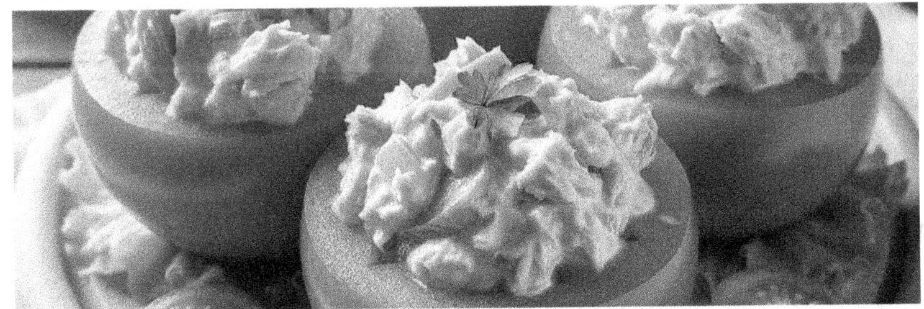

**Ingredients:**

- 4 large tomatoes
- 1 can (5 ounces) tuna in water, drained
- 2 tablespoons mayonnaise
- Salt and pepper to taste
- 2 tablespoons chopped parsley (optional for garnish)

**Preparation:**

1. Cut the tops off the tomatoes and carefully scoop out the seeds and inner flesh to create a hollow shell. Lightly salt the inside and place them upside down on a paper towel to drain any excess moisture.
2. In a bowl, mix the drained tuna with mayonnaise. Season with salt and pepper according to taste.
3. Fill the hollowed tomatoes with the tuna salad mixture.
4. Garnish with chopped parsley if desired.

**Cooking Time:** No cooking required; preparation time is about 15 minutes.

**Nutritional Values** (approximate per serving):

- Calories: 150
- Protein: 13g
- Carbohydrates: 8g
- Fat: 7g
- Fiber: 2g
- Sugar: 4g

**Rating:** ★★★★★

Tuna Salad Stuffed Tomatoes offer a refreshing and nutritious twist on the classic tuna salad. Perfect for a light lunch or as a healthy appetizer, this dish combines the succulence of fresh tomatoes with the savory flavors of tuna salad, creating a meal that's not only satisfying but also visually appealing.

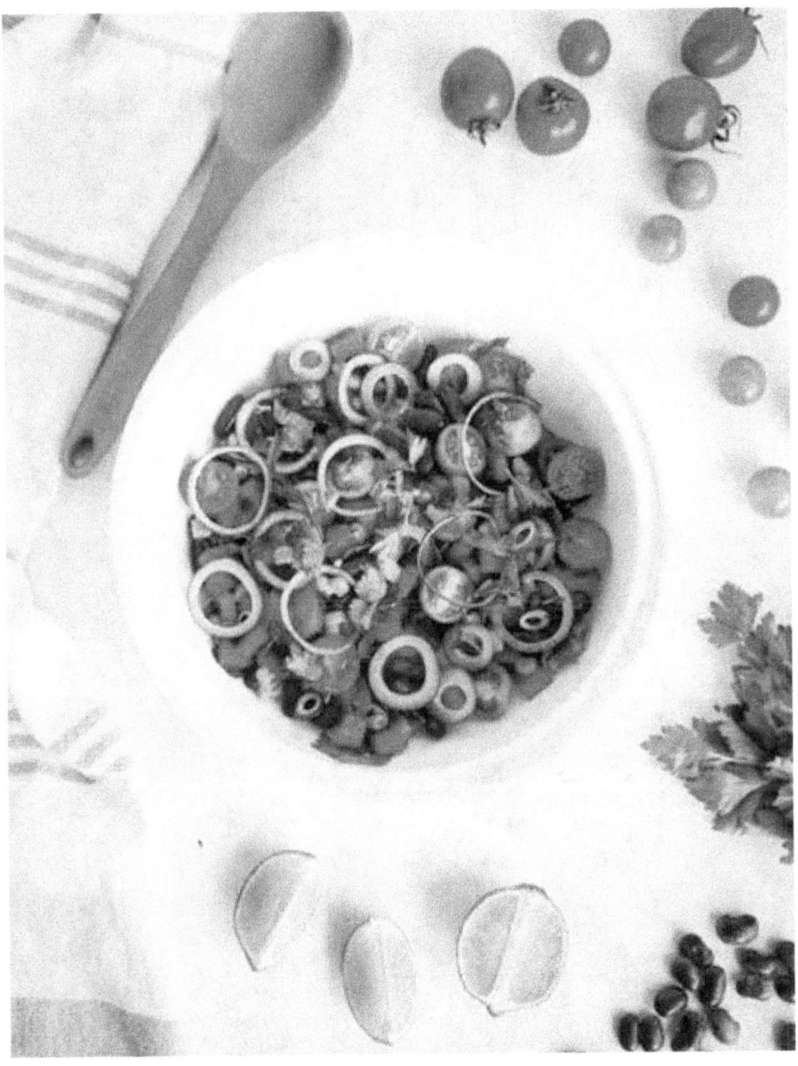

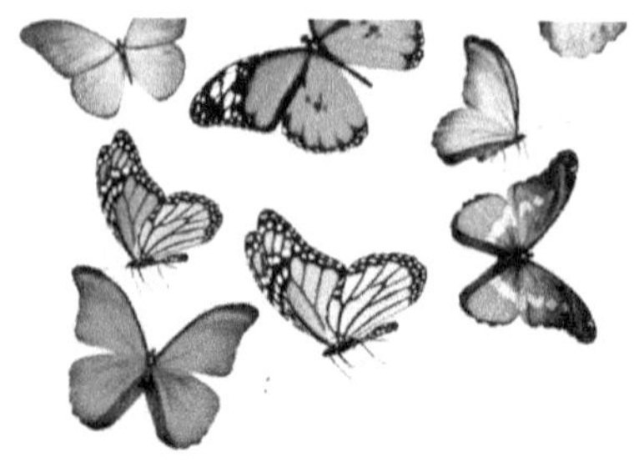

"Remember, small changes lead to big victories. Each healthy choice you make is a victory in your post-surgery journey."

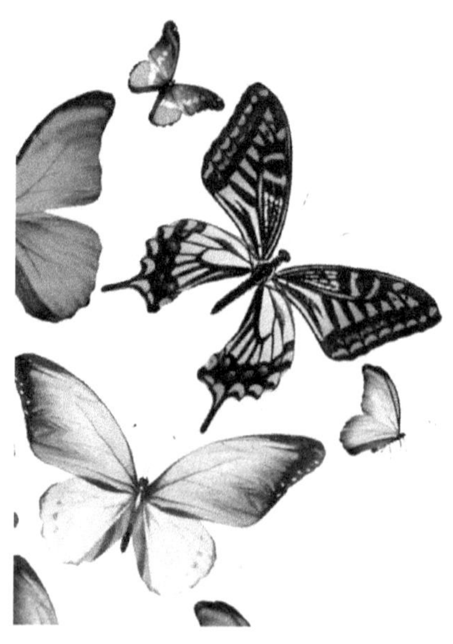

# Dinner

Dinner is your opportunity to unwind and nourish your body after a day's activities, especially crucial after gastric sleeve surgery when your body is adapting to new dietary changes. Our dinner recipes are thoughtfully designed to be both satisfying and gentle on your new stomach. With only five ingredients, these dishes are simple to prepare, ensuring that you can enjoy a nutritious meal without the hassle of complex recipes or a long list of ingredients. Embrace these easy-to-make, delicious dinners as you continue on your journey to a healthier lifestyle, enjoying the flavors and textures that make each meal a delightful experience.

## Baked Salmon with Asparagus

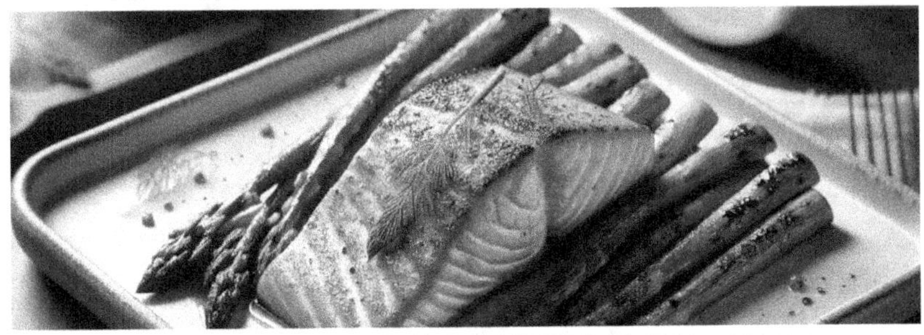

## Ingredients:

- 2 salmon fillets (6 ounces each)
- 1 bunch asparagus, trimmed
- 2 tablespoons olive oil
- Salt and pepper to taste
- Lemon wedges (for serving)

## Preparation:

1. Preheat the oven to 400°F (200°C).
2. Arrange the asparagus in a single layer on a baking sheet. Drizzle with 1 tablespoon of olive oil and season with salt and pepper.
3. Place the salmon fillets on top of the asparagus. Drizzle the remaining olive oil over the salmon and season with salt and pepper.
4. Bake in the preheated oven for about 15-20 minutes, or until the salmon is cooked through and flakes easily with a fork.
5. Serve hot with lemon wedges on the side.

**Cooking Time:** 20 minutes

**Nutritional Values** (approximate per serving):

- Calories: 300
- Protein: 23g
- Carbohydrates: 5g
- Fat: 22g
- Fiber: 2g
- Sugar: 2g

**Rating: ★★★★★**

Baked Salmon with Asparagus is a simple, healthy, and flavorful dinner option. The rich omega-3 fatty acids in salmon combined with the fiber in asparagus make this dish not only delicious but also incredibly nutritious. Perfect for a quick weeknight dinner or a special occasion, this meal is sure to satisfy.

## Turkey Meatballs with Zucchini Noodles

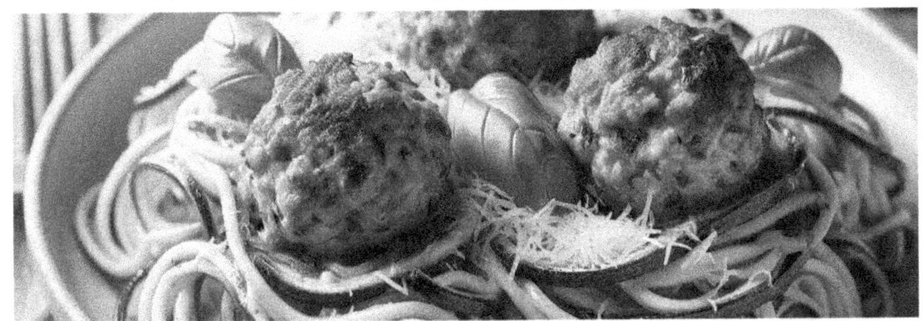

**Ingredients:**

- 1 pound ground turkey
- 2 zucchinis, spiralized into noodles
- 1/4 cup breadcrumbs (use almond meal for low-carb option)
- 1/4 cup grated Parmesan cheese
- Salt and pepper to taste

**Preparation:**

1. In a bowl, combine the ground turkey, breadcrumbs, grated Parmesan cheese, salt, and pepper. Mix until well incorporated.

2. Form the mixture into meatballs, about 1 to 1.5 inches in diameter.

3. In a non-stick skillet, cook the turkey meatballs over medium heat, turning occasionally, until they are browned on all sides and cooked through (about 12-15 minutes).

4. In the same skillet, add the zucchini noodles and sauté for 2-3 minutes until tender.

5. Serve the turkey meatballs on top of the zucchini noodles.

**Cooking Time:** 20 minutes

**Nutritional Values** (approximate per serving):

- Calories: 350
- Protein: 30g
- Carbohydrates: 10g
- Fat: 21g
- Fiber: 2g
- Sugar: 4g

**Rating:** ★★★★★

Turkey Meatballs with Zucchini Noodles offer a lean and satisfying dinner option. The turkey meatballs are seasoned to perfection and pair wonderfully with fresh zucchini noodles, providing a low-carb alternative to traditional pasta. This dish is not only healthy but also bursting with flavor, making it a great choice for a hearty, guilt-free meal.

## Salsa Chicken and Rice Casserole

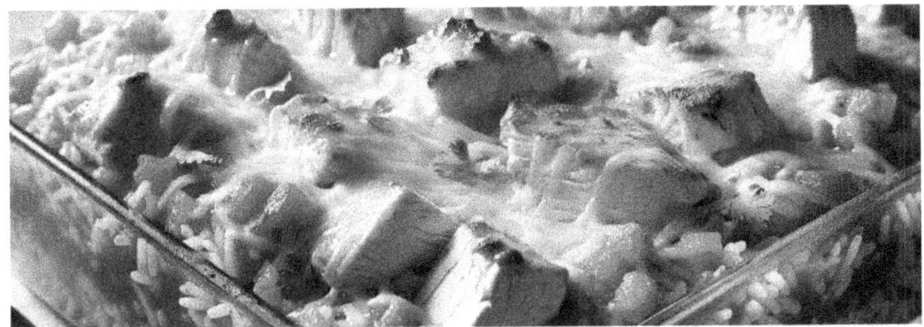

**Ingredients:**

- 2 cups cooked chicken breast, shredded
- 1 cup cooked white rice
- 1 cup salsa (choose your preferred spice level)
- 1 cup shredded cheddar cheese
- 1 teaspoon chili powder
- Salt and pepper to taste

**Preparation:**

1. Preheat the oven to 350°F (175°C).
2. In a large mixing bowl, combine the cooked chicken, cooked rice, salsa, half of the shredded cheddar cheese, chili powder, salt, and pepper.
3. Transfer the mixture into a baking dish and spread it evenly.
4. Top with the remaining shredded cheddar cheese.
5. Bake in the preheated oven for about 20-25 minutes, or until the cheese is melted and bubbly.
6. Optionally, broil for a minute or two to achieve a golden, crispy top.

**Cooking Time:** 25 minutes

**Nutritional Values** (approximate per serving):

- Calories: 350
- Protein: 30g
- Carbohydrates: 25g
- Fat: 14g
- Fiber: 2g
- Sugar: 2g

**Rating:** ★★★★★

Salsa Chicken and Rice Casserole is a comforting and flavorful dinner option. It's a perfect way to use up leftover chicken and rice while creating a delicious, cheesy casserole. The combination of salsa and spices adds a delightful kick to this dish, making it a family favorite that's both easy to prepare and satisfying to eat.

## Pork Tenderloin with Roasted Brussels Sprouts

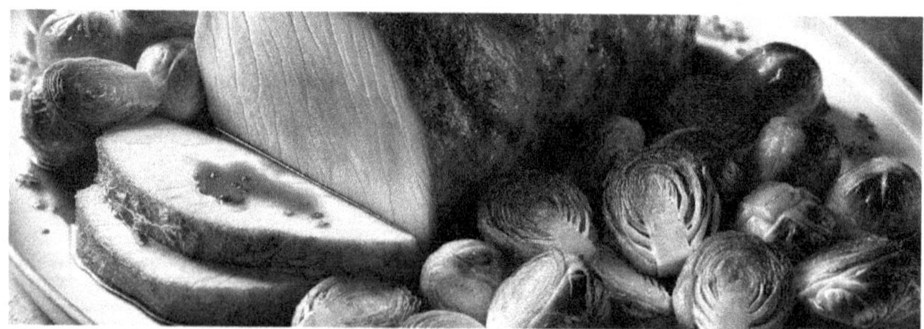

**Ingredients:**

- 2 pork tenderloin fillets (6-8 ounces each)
- 2 cups Brussels sprouts, trimmed and halved
- 2 tablespoons olive oil

- Salt and pepper to taste
- 1 teaspoon dried thyme

**Preparation:**

1. Preheat the oven to 425°F (220°C).

2. In a mixing bowl, toss the Brussels sprouts with 1 tablespoon of olive oil, salt, pepper, and dried thyme.

3. Place the pork tenderloin fillets on a baking sheet. Brush them with the remaining olive oil and season with salt and pepper.

4. Spread the seasoned Brussels sprouts around the pork on the baking sheet.

5. Roast in the preheated oven for 20-25 minutes or until the pork reaches an internal temperature of 145°F (63°C) and the Brussels sprouts are tender.

**Cooking Time:** 25 minutes

**Nutritional Values** (approximate per serving):

- Calories: 350
- Fat: 20g
- Protein: 30g
- Fiber: 4g
- Carbohydrates: 10g
- Sugar: 2g

**Rating:** ★★★★★

Pork Tenderloin with Roasted Brussels Sprouts is a delightful and wholesome dinner option. The tender pork pairs perfectly with the caramelized Brussels sprouts, and the dried thyme adds a fragrant touch. This dish is not only delicious but also provides a balanced meal that's easy to prepare, making it a fantastic choice for a satisfying dinner.

## Shrimp Stir-Fry with Mixed Vegetables

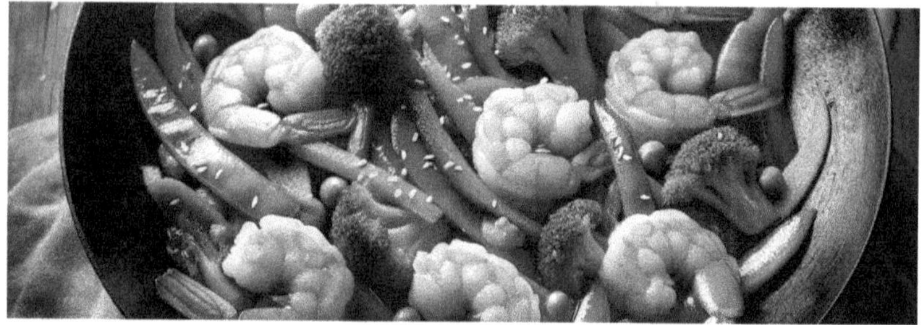

**Ingredients:**

- 1-pound large shrimp, peeled and deveined
- 2 cups mixed vegetables (broccoli, bell peppers, snap peas, carrots)
- 2 tablespoons low-sodium soy sauce
- 1 tablespoon sesame oil
- 1 teaspoon ginger, minced
- Salt and pepper to taste

**Preparation:**

1. In a wok or large skillet, heat the sesame oil over medium-high heat.

2. Add the minced ginger and stir-fry for about 30 seconds until fragrant.

3. Add the shrimp and cook for 2-3 minutes until they start to turn pink.

4. Add the mixed vegetables and continue to stir-fry for another 3-4 minutes until they are tender-crisp.

5. Drizzle with soy sauce and season with salt and pepper. Stir to combine and cook for an additional 1-2 minutes.

6. Serve hot.

**Cooking Time:** 15 minutes

**Nutritional Values** (approximate per serving):

- Calories: 250
- Protein: 30g
- Carbohydrates: 10g
- Fat: 8g
- Fiber: 4g
- Sugar: 3g

**Rating: ★★★★★**

Shrimp Stir-Fry with Mixed Vegetables is a quick and healthy dinner option. Packed with protein and vibrant vegetables, it offers a burst of flavors and textures. The ginger and soy sauce add a savory touch to this dish, making it a satisfying and nutritious choice for a delicious weeknight dinner.

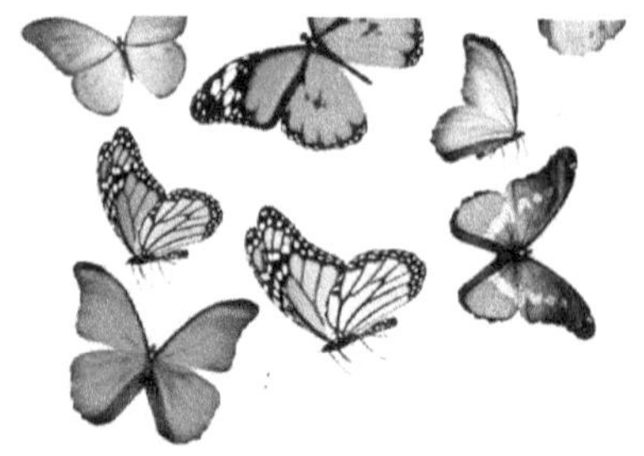

"You're not alone on this path. With every spoonful, remember there's a community cheering you on towards your goals."

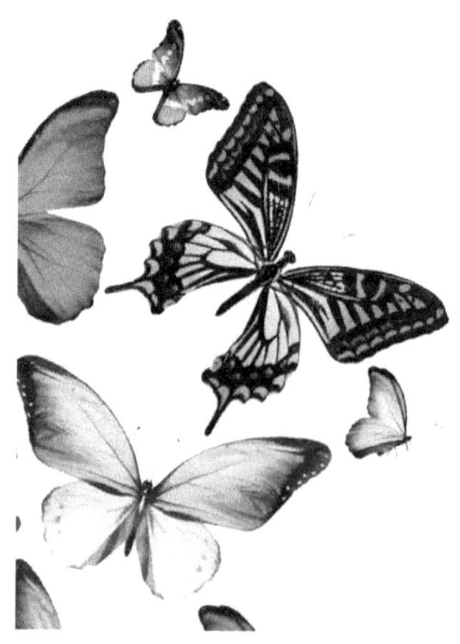

# Snacks and Sides

Snacks and sides play a crucial role in keeping your energy levels stable throughout the day while maintaining a balanced diet after gastric sleeve surgery. Our snack and side recipes are designed to be easy to prepare and satisfying to your taste buds. With just five ingredients, these dishes offer a variety of flavors and textures, making them a perfect complement to your main meals. These recipes will keep your cravings in check and your stomach happy. Enjoy these simple yet delightful snacks and sides to make your post-surgery journey enjoyable and nutritious.

## Cucumber and Hummus Bites

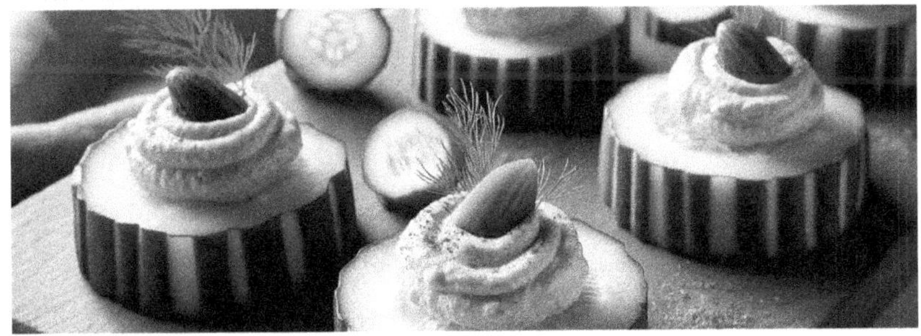

**Ingredients:**

- 1 cucumber, sliced into rounds
- 1/2 cup hummus (store-bought or homemade)
- Cherry tomatoes for garnish (optional)
- Fresh parsley for garnish (optional)
- Paprika for garnish (optional)

**Preparation:**

1. Slice the cucumber into rounds, about 1/2 inch thick.
2. Using a small spoon or melon baller, scoop out a small portion of the center of each cucumber slice to create a little well.
3. Fill each well with a dollop of hummus.
4. Garnish with a halved cherry tomato, fresh parsley, and a sprinkle of paprika if desired.
5. Serve chilled.

**Cooking Time:** No cooking required; preparation time is about 10 minutes.

**Nutritional Values** (approximate per serving, 4 cucumber rounds with hummus):

- Calories: 50
- Protein: 2g
- Carbohydrates: 5g
- Fat: 3g
- Fiber: 1g
- Sugar: 1g

**Rating: ★★★★★**

Cucumber and Hummus Bites are a refreshing and healthy snack or side option. The cool crunch of cucumber pairs perfectly with the creamy hummus, creating a satisfying and hydrating combination. With minimal preparation, these bites are not only delicious but also visually appealing, making them a great addition to any meal or a quick, guilt-free snack.

## Roasted Chickpeas

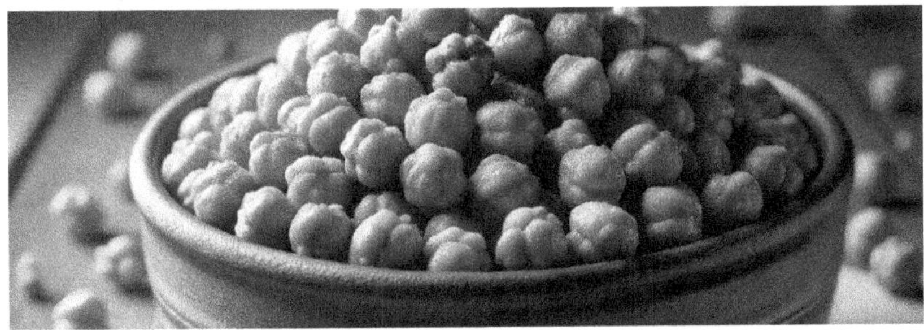

**Ingredients:**

- 1 can (15 ounces) chickpeas (garbanzo beans), drained and rinsed
- 2 tablespoons olive oil
- 1 teaspoon paprika
- 1/2 teaspoon cumin
- Salt and pepper to taste

**Preparation:**

1. Preheat the oven to 400°F (200°C).
2. Rinse and drain the chickpeas, then pat them dry with a paper towel.

3. In a bowl, toss the chickpeas with olive oil, paprika, cumin, salt, and pepper until they are well coated.

4. Spread the seasoned chickpeas in a single layer on a baking sheet.

5. Roast in the preheated oven for 25-30 minutes, or until they are crispy and golden brown, shaking the pan occasionally for even cooking.

6. Let cool before serving.

**Cooking Time:** 30 minutes

**Nutritional Values** (approximate per serving):

- Calories: 150
- Protein: 5g
- Carbohydrates: 15g
- Fat: 8g
- Fiber: 4g
- Sugar: 0g

**Rating:** ★★★★★

Roasted Chickpeas are a crunchy and satisfying snack or side dish. They are packed with fiber and protein, making them a nutritious and flavorful option. The combination of spices adds a delightful kick to this snack, making it an ideal choice for those looking for a guilt-free, crunchy treat.

## Sweet Potato Fries

**Ingredients:**

- 2 large sweet potatoes, peeled and cut into fries
- 2 tablespoons olive oil
- 1 teaspoon paprika
- 1/2 teaspoon garlic powder
- Salt and pepper to taste

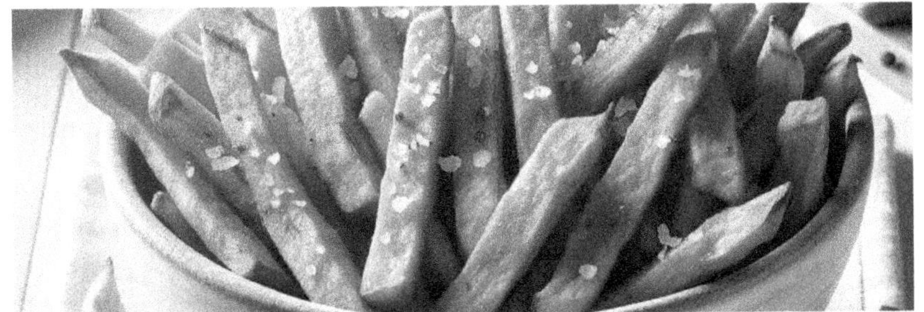

**Preparation:**

1. Preheat the oven to 425°F (220°C).
2. In a large bowl, toss the sweet potato fries with olive oil, paprika, garlic powder, salt, and pepper until they are evenly coated.
3. Spread the seasoned sweet potato fries in a single layer on a baking sheet.
4. Roast in the preheated oven for 20-25 minutes, flipping halfway through, until they are crispy and golden brown.
5. Serve hot.

**Cooking Time:** 25 minutes

**Nutritional Values** (approximate per serving):

- Calories: 150
- Protein: 2g
- Carbohydrates: 28g
- Fat: 4g

- Fiber: 4g
- Sugar: 6g

**Rating: ★★★★★**

Sweet Potato Fries are a delightful and nutritious snack or side dish. They offer the perfect combination of sweetness and crispiness, making them a healthier alternative to traditional french fries. The paprika and garlic powder add a burst of flavor to these fries, making them a tasty and guilt-free treat.

## Garlic Parmesan Green Beans

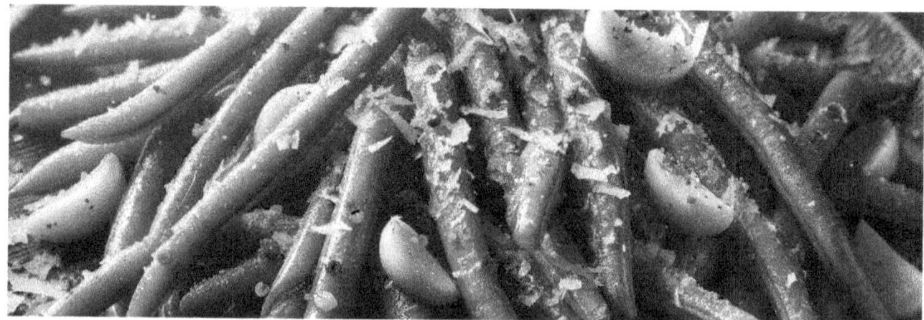

**Ingredients:**

- 1-pound fresh green beans, trimmed
- 2 tablespoons olive oil
- 2 cloves garlic, minced
- 1/4 cup grated Parmesan cheese
- Salt and pepper to taste

**Preparation:**

1. In a large skillet, heat olive oil over medium-high heat.
2. Add minced garlic and sauté for about 1 minute until fragrant.

3. Add the green beans to the skillet and stir-fry for 5-7 minutes until they are tender-crisp.

4. Sprinkle with grated Parmesan cheese and continue to cook for an additional 2-3 minutes, or until the cheese is melted.

5. Season with salt and pepper according to taste.

**Cooking Time:** 10 minutes

**Nutritional Values** (approximate per serving):

- Calories: 100
- Protein: 3g
- Carbohydrates: 7g
- Fat: 7g
- Fiber: 3g
- Sugar: 2g

**Rating:** ★★★★★

Garlic Parmesan Green Beans are a flavorful and nutritious side dish. The combination of garlic, Parmesan cheese, and perfectly sautéed green beans creates a dish that's not only delicious but also visually appealing.

## Caprese Salad Skewers

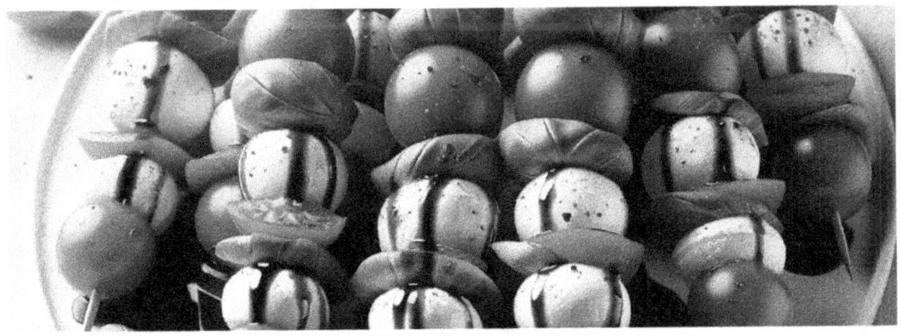

**Ingredients:**

- Cherry tomatoes
- Fresh mozzarella cheese balls
- Fresh basil leaves
- Balsamic glaze (store-bought or homemade)
- Wooden skewers

**Preparation:**

1. Take a wooden skewer and thread on a cherry tomato.
2. Follow with a mozzarella cheese ball and a fresh basil leaf.
3. Repeat the pattern until the skewer is filled.
4. Drizzle with balsamic glaze just before serving.

**Cooking Time:** No cooking required; preparation time is about 10 minutes.

**Nutritional Values** (approximate per serving):

- Calories: 50
- Protein: 2g
- Carbohydrates: 2g
- Fat: 3g
- Fiber: 0g
- Sugar: 1g

**Rating:** ★★★★★

Caprese Salad Skewers are a delightful and visually appealing snack or side dish. The combination of fresh tomatoes, creamy mozzarella, and fragrant basil, drizzled with balsamic glaze, creates a burst of flavors and textures.

# Desserts

Desserts are a great way to fulfill your sweet appetite while following a bariatric diet. Our dessert recipes are meticulously designed to be both decadent and portion-controlled, allowing you to enjoy a treat without jeopardizing your nutritional objectives. These desserts require only five ingredients and are a guilt-free way to conclude your dinner on a sweet note. Accept these delightful and healthy dessert selections to make your post-surgery meal experience full and pleasurable.

## Greek Yogurt with Honey and Walnuts

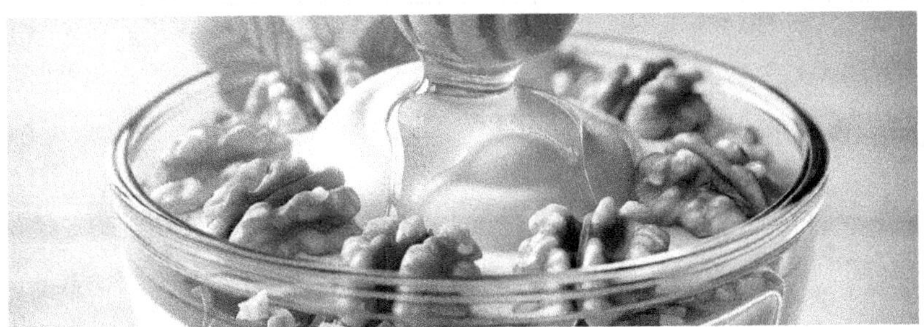

**Ingredients:**

- 1 cup Greek yogurt
- 2 tablespoons honey

- 1/4 cup walnuts, chopped
- Fresh berries for garnish (optional)
- Mint leaves for garnish (optional)

**Preparation:**

1. Spoon Greek yogurt into a serving bowl or glass.
2. Drizzle honey over the yogurt.
3. Sprinkle chopped walnuts on top.
4. Garnish with fresh berries and mint leaves if desired.
5. Serve chilled.

**Cooking Time:** No cooking required; preparation time is about 5 minutes.

**Nutritional Values** (approximate per serving):

- Calories: 250
- Protein: 15g
- Carbohydrates: 20g
- Fat: 13g
- Fiber: 1g
- Sugar: 17g

**Rating:** ★★★★★

Greek Yogurt with Honey and Walnuts is a simple and satisfying dessert. The creamy Greek yogurt pairs wonderfully with the sweetness of honey and the crunch of walnuts. It's a delightful treat that offers a balance of flavors and textures, making it a perfect way to end your meal on a healthy and delicious note.

# Baked Apples with Cinnamon

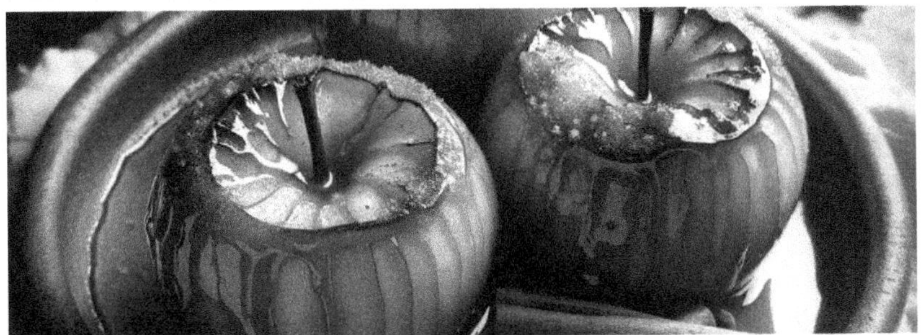

## Ingredients:

- 2 apples, cored and halved
- 1 teaspoon cinnamon
- 1 tablespoon honey
- 1 tablespoon chopped nuts (e.g., almonds, pecans)
- Greek yogurt or vanilla ice cream (optional for serving)

## Preparation:

1. Preheat the oven to 375°F (190°C).
2. Place the apple halves, cut side up, on a baking sheet or in a baking dish.
3. Sprinkle cinnamon evenly over the apples.
4. Drizzle honey over the apples and sprinkle with chopped nuts.
5. Bake in the preheated oven for 20-25 minutes, or until the apples are tender and slightly caramelized.
6. Serve warm, optionally with a dollop of Greek yogurt or a scoop of vanilla ice cream.

**Cooking Time:** 25 minutes

**Nutritional Values** (approximate per serving, without optional toppings):

- Calories: 150
- Protein: 1g
- Carbohydrates: 40g
- Fat: 1g
- Fiber: 5g
- Sugar: 30g

**Rating:** ★★★★★

Baked Apples with Cinnamon is a warm and comforting dessert. The natural sweetness of the apples combines with the warmth of cinnamon and the richness of honey to create a delightful treat. The addition of chopped nuts adds a satisfying crunch. It's a healthier dessert option that's perfect for satisfying your sweet cravings without the guilt.

## Berry and Ricotta Cheese Parfait

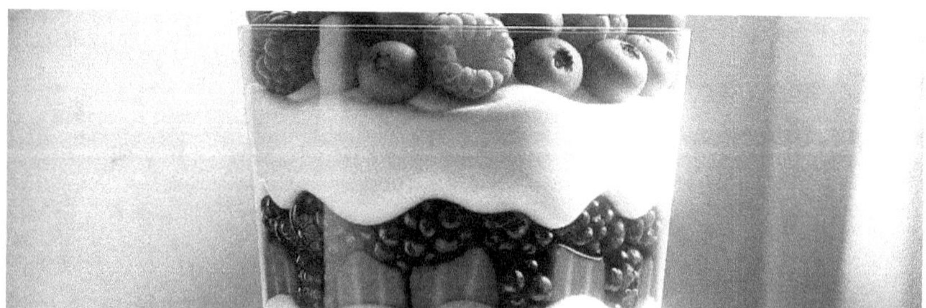

**Ingredients:**

- 1 cup fresh mixed berries (e.g., strawberries, blueberries, raspberries)
- 1/2 cup ricotta cheese
- 1 tablespoon honey
- 2 tablespoons granola
- Fresh mint leaves for garnish (optional)

## Preparation:

1. In a serving glass or bowl, layer half of the mixed berries.
2. Spoon half of the ricotta cheese over the berries.
3. Drizzle with honey.
4. Add half of the granola.
5. Repeat the layers with the remaining ingredients.
6. Garnish with fresh mint leaves if desired.
7. Serve chilled.

**Cooking Time:** No cooking required; preparation time is about 5 minutes.

**Nutritional Values** (approximate per serving):

- Calories: 250
- Protein: 10g
- Carbohydrates: 30g
- Fat: 10g
- Fiber: 4g
- Sugar: 16g

**Rating:** ★★★★★

Berry and Ricotta Cheese Parfait is a refreshing and wholesome dessert. The combination of fresh berries, creamy ricotta cheese, honey, and granola creates a harmonious blend of flavors and textures. It's a delightful and nutritious way to satisfy your dessert cravings while keeping your diet on track.

## Chocolate Avocado Mousse

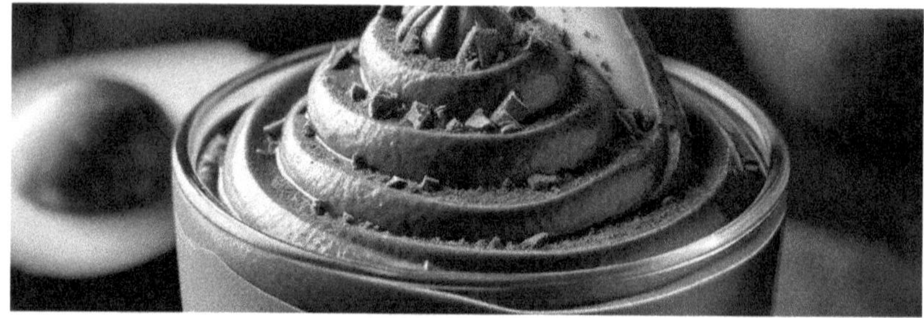

**Ingredients:**

- 2 ripe avocados
- 1/4 cup unsweetened cocoa powder
- 1/4 cup honey or maple syrup
- 1 teaspoon vanilla extract
- A pinch of salt

**Preparation:**

1. Scoop the flesh of the ripe avocados into a food processor.
2. Add cocoa powder, honey (or maple syrup), vanilla extract, and a pinch of salt.
3. Blend until smooth and creamy, scraping down the sides as needed.
4. Transfer the mousse to serving bowls or glasses.
5. Refrigerate for at least 30 minutes before serving.

6. Optionally, garnish with berries or shaved chocolate.

**Cooking Time:** No cooking required; preparation time is about 10 minutes.

**Nutritional Values** (approximate per serving):

- Calories: 200
- Protein: 3g
- Carbohydrates: 20g
- Fat: 15g
- Fiber: 7g
- Sugar: 11g

**Rating: ★★★★★**

Chocolate Avocado Mousse is a creamy and decadent dessert with a healthy twist. The richness of ripe avocados blends perfectly with cocoa powder and a touch of sweetness. It's a guilt-free way to enjoy the indulgence of chocolate mousse while adding the nutritional benefits of avocados. This dessert is sure to satisfy your chocolate cravings in a wholesome manner.

## Peanut Butter Banana Ice Cream

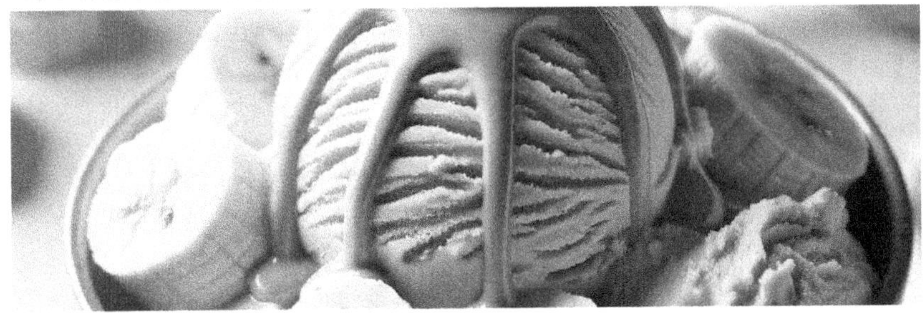

**Ingredients:**

- 2 ripe bananas, peeled and sliced
- 2 tablespoons peanut butter (unsweetened)
- 1/2 teaspoon vanilla extract
- A pinch of salt
- Optional toppings (e.g., chopped nuts, dark chocolate chips)

**Preparation:**

1. Arrange the banana slices on a baking sheet and freeze until solid (about 2 hours).
2. In a food processor, combine the frozen banana slices, peanut butter, vanilla extract, and a pinch of salt.
3. Blend until smooth and creamy, scraping down the sides as needed.
4. Transfer the ice cream to a bowl and freeze for an additional 30 minutes if a firmer texture is desired.
5. Optionally, garnish with chopped nuts or dark chocolate chips before serving.

**Cooking Time:** No cooking required; preparation time is about 10 minutes (excluding freezing time).

**Nutritional Values** (approximate per serving, without optional toppings):

- Calories: 200
- Protein: 4g

- Carbohydrates: 28g
- Fat: 9g
- Fiber: 3g
- Sugar: 14g

**Rating: ★★★★★**

Peanut Butter Banana Ice Cream is a creamy and satisfying dessert with a natural sweetness. The combination of frozen bananas and peanut butter creates a delightful flavor that resembles traditional ice cream. It's a guilt-free and dairy-free alternative to satisfy your ice cream cravings, making it a perfect treat for any time of the day.

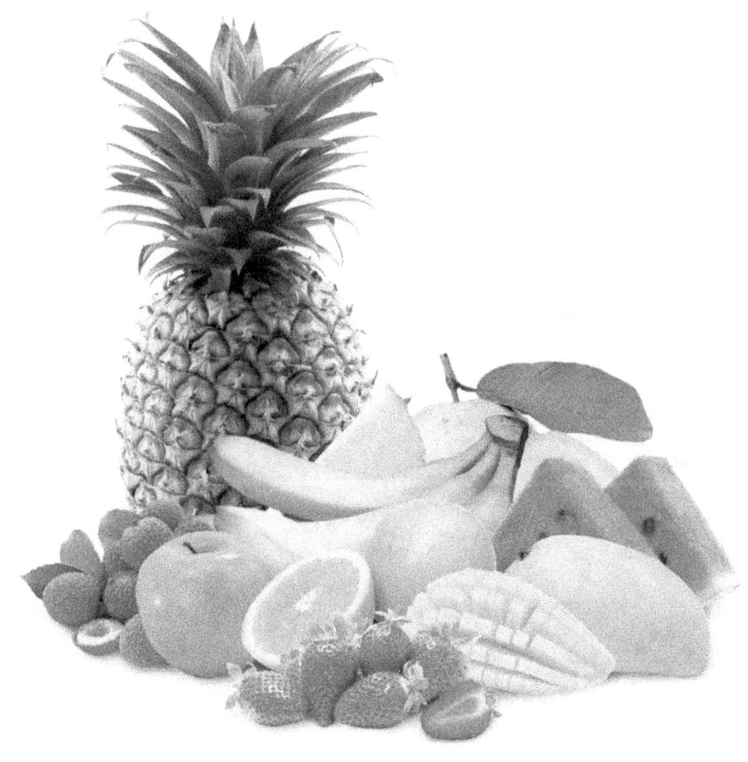

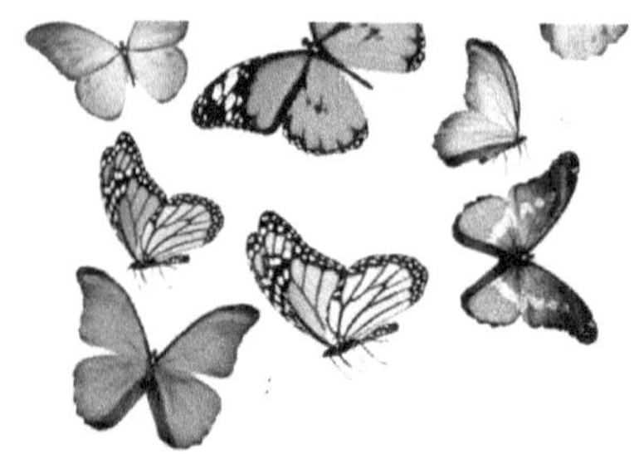

"Nourish your body, nourish your soul. Let food be your ally in healing, not just a necessity."

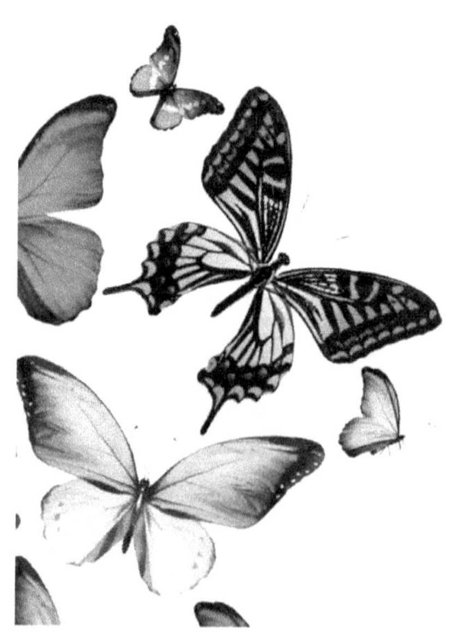

# Meat and Poultry

Meat and poultry dishes are important sources of protein in a bariatric diet. Our meat and poultry dishes are tasty, easy to make, and tailored to your nutritional needs following gastric sleeve surgery. With only five ingredients, these recipes are a tasty and protein-rich addition to your meals. Enjoy these easy yet delicious meat and poultry recipes to make your post-surgery meal more fun and nutritious.

## Lemon Herb Chicken Breast

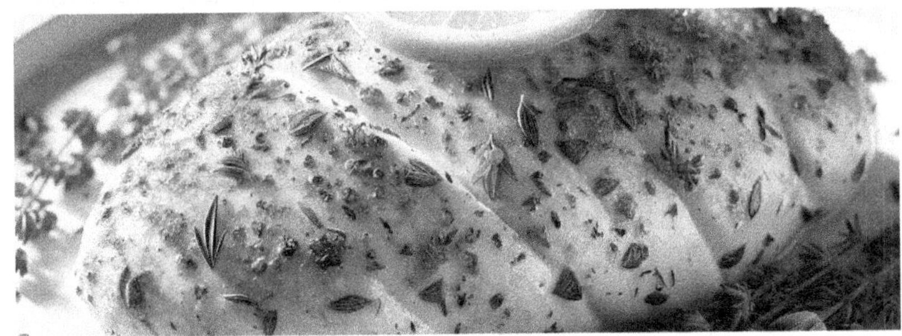

**Ingredients:**

- 2 boneless, skinless chicken breasts
- Juice of 1 lemon
- 2 tablespoons olive oil
- 1 teaspoon dried herbs (e.g., thyme, rosemary, oregano)
- Salt and pepper to taste

**Preparation:**

1. In a bowl, combine the lemon juice, olive oil, dried herbs, salt, and pepper to create a marinade.
2. Place the chicken breasts in a resealable plastic bag or a shallow dish and pour the marinade over them.
3. Seal the bag or cover the dish and refrigerate for at least 30 minutes (or up to 24 hours for a stronger flavor).
4. Preheat a grill or skillet over medium-high heat.
5. Grill or pan-fry the chicken breasts for about 6-7 minutes per side, or until they are cooked through and have grill marks.
6. Let the chicken rest for a few minutes before serving.

**Cooking Time:** 15 minutes (plus marinating time)

**Nutritional Values** (approximate per serving):

- Calories: 200
- Protein: 25g
- Carbohydrates: 2g
- Fat: 10g
- Fiber: 0g
- Sugar: 0g

**Rating:** ★★★★★

Lemon Herb Chicken Breast is a flavorful and protein-rich dish. The combination of zesty lemon and aromatic herbs infuses the chicken with a delightful taste. Whether grilled or pan-fried, this dish is quick and easy to prepare, making it a perfect choice for a nutritious and tasty meal.

## Beef and Broccoli

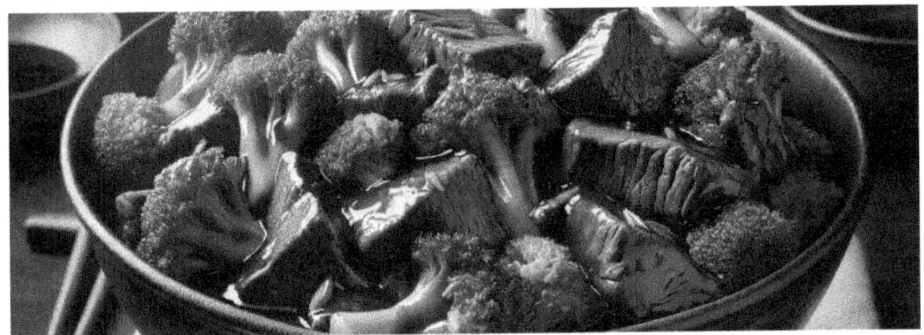

**Ingredients:**

- 1 pound beef sirloin, thinly sliced

- 2 cups broccoli florets

- 2 tablespoons low-sodium soy sauce

- 1 tablespoon olive oil

- 1 teaspoon garlic, minced

- Salt and pepper to taste

**Preparation:**

1. In a bowl, marinate the sliced beef with soy sauce, minced garlic, salt, and pepper. Let it sit for 10-15 minutes.

2. Heat olive oil in a skillet or wok over high heat.

3. Add the marinated beef and stir-fry for 2-3 minutes until it's no longer pink. Remove from the skillet and set aside.

4. In the same skillet, add the broccoli florets and stir-fry for 3-4 minutes until they are tender-crisp.

5. Return the cooked beef to the skillet and stir-fry for an additional 1-2 minutes to combine all ingredients.

6. Serve hot.

**Cooking Time:** 15 minutes

**Nutritional Values** (approximate per serving):

- Calories: 250
- Protein: 25g
- Carbohydrates: 8g
- Fat: 12g
- Fiber: 3g
- Sugar: 2g

**Rating:** ★★★★★

Beef and Broccoli is a savory and satisfying dish that's quick to prepare. The tender beef and crisp broccoli are coated in a flavorful soy sauce and garlic mixture. It's a balanced meal that provides protein and vegetables in one delicious plate. This recipe offers a delightful combination of textures and tastes, making it a favorite for those looking for a simple and tasty meal option.

## Turkey Burger Patties

**Ingredients:**

- 1 pound ground turkey
- 1/4 cup breadcrumbs (preferably whole wheat)
- 1/4 cup grated Parmesan cheese
- 1 teaspoon dried Italian seasoning
- Salt and pepper to taste

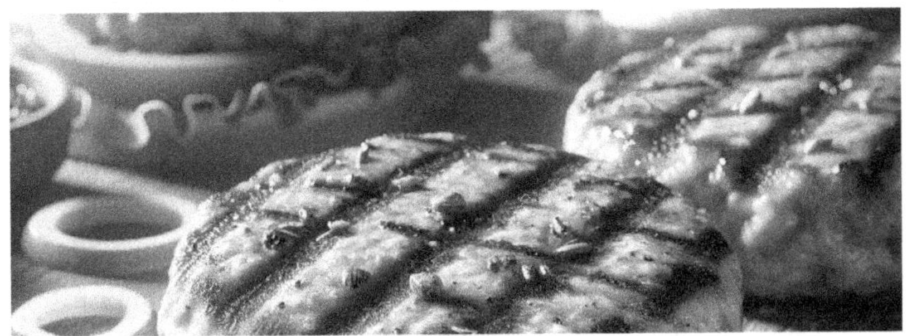

**Preparation:**

1. In a bowl, combine the ground turkey, breadcrumbs, grated Parmesan cheese, dried Italian seasoning, salt, and pepper.
2. Mix the ingredients until well combined.
3. Divide the mixture into 4 equal portions and shape them into burger patties.
4. Preheat a grill or skillet over medium-high heat.
5. Grill or pan-fry the turkey burger patties for about 5-6 minutes per side, or until they are cooked through and have reached an internal temperature of 165°F (74°C).
6. Serve on whole wheat buns with your favorite toppings.

**Cooking Time:** 15 minutes

**Nutritional Values** (approximate per patty, excluding bun and toppings):

- Calories: 180
- Protein: 21g
- Carbohydrates: 5g
- Fat: 8g
- Fiber: 1g
- Sugar: 0g

**Rating:** ★★★★☆

Turkey Burger Patties are a lean and flavorful alternative to traditional beef burgers. Packed with protein and seasoned with Italian herbs and Parmesan cheese, these patties offer a delicious and satisfying meal. Whether grilled or pan-fried, they are quick to cook and make for a nutritious option for your bariatric diet.

## Balsamic Glazed Pork Chops

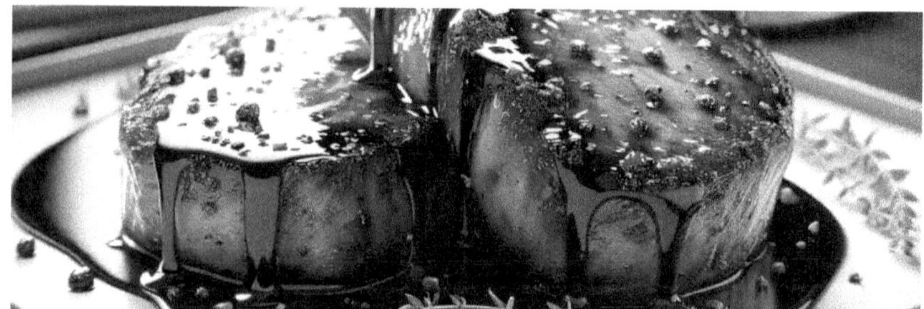

**Ingredients:**

- 4 boneless pork chops
- 1/4 cup balsamic vinegar
- 2 tablespoons honey
- 1 teaspoon garlic, minced
- Salt and pepper to taste

## Preparation:

1. In a bowl, whisk together balsamic vinegar, honey, minced garlic, salt, and pepper to create the glaze.
2. Brush both sides of the pork chops with the glaze.
3. Preheat a grill or skillet over medium-high heat.
4. Grill or pan-fry the pork chops for about 4-5 minutes per side, or until they are cooked through and have reached an internal temperature of 145°F (63°C).
5. Brush with additional glaze during cooking for extra flavor.
6. Serve hot.

**Cooking Time:** 15 minutes

**Nutritional Values** (approximate per pork chop):

- Calories: 200
- Protein: 25g
- Carbohydrates: 7g
- Fat: 7g
- Fiber: 0g
- Sugar: 6g

**Rating:** ★★★★★

Balsamic Glazed Pork Chops are a succulent and tangy dish. The sweet and savory balsamic glaze adds a burst of flavor to tender pork chops. Whether grilled or pan-fried, these chops are quick and easy to prepare, making them a delightful addition to your meal. The combination of honey and balsamic vinegar creates a harmonious balance of flavors that will satisfy your taste buds.

## Chicken and Vegetable Kebabs

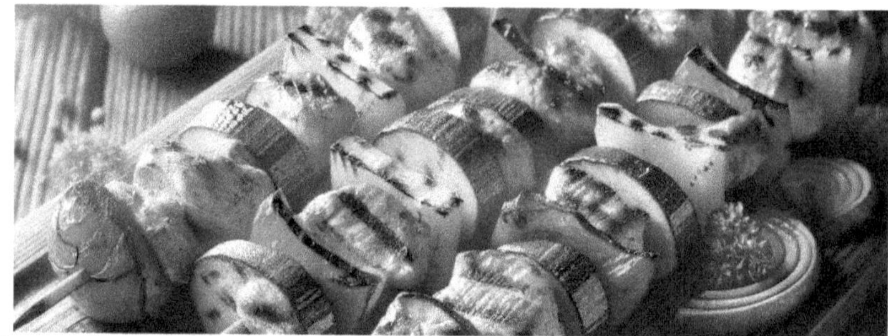

**Ingredients:**

- 1-pound boneless, skinless chicken breast, cut into cubes
- Assorted vegetables (e.g., bell peppers, onions, zucchini), cut into chunks
- 2 tablespoons olive oil
- 1 teaspoon dried herbs (e.g., oregano, thyme)
- Salt and pepper to taste

**Preparation:**

1. In a bowl, combine the chicken cubes, assorted vegetables, olive oil, dried herbs, salt, and pepper. Toss until well coated.
2. Thread the chicken and vegetable pieces onto skewers, alternating between chicken and vegetables.
3. Preheat a grill to medium-high heat.
4. Grill the kebabs for about 10-12 minutes, turning occasionally, until the chicken is cooked through and the vegetables are tender.
5. Serve hot.

**Cooking Time:** 15 minutes

**Nutritional Values** (approximate per serving):

- Calories: 250
- Protein: 25g
- Carbohydrates: 5g
- Fat: 14g
- Fiber: 2g
- Sugar: 2g

**Rating:** ★★★★★

Chicken and Vegetable Kebabs are a delightful and balanced meal option. These kebabs are not only visually appealing but also packed with flavor. The combination of marinated chicken and grilled vegetables creates a satisfying and nutritious dish. Whether served as a main course or party appetizer, these kebabs are a crowd-pleaser that's simple to prepare and perfect for your bariatric diet.

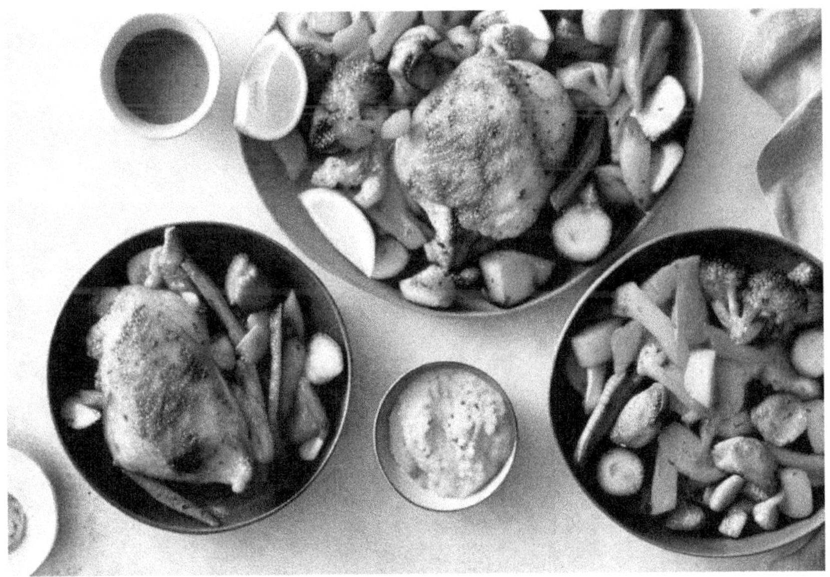

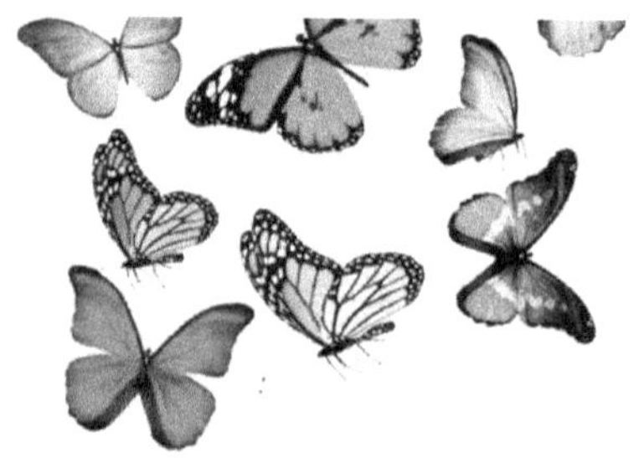

"Your willpower is stronger than any craving. When you choose health, you choose a future filled with possibilities."

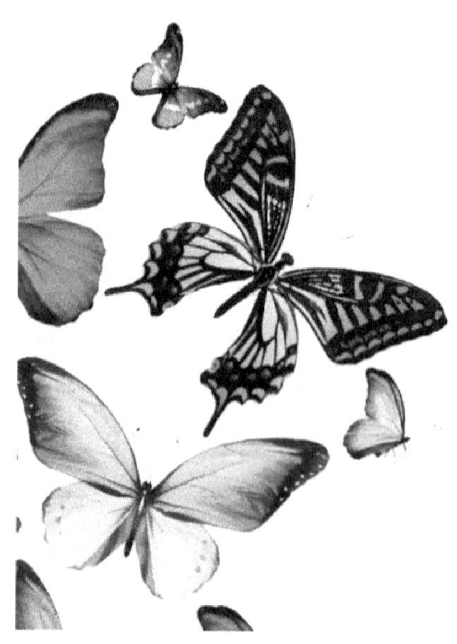

# Soups

Soups are a pleasant and healthy addition to your bariatric diet. Our soup recipes are carefully created to deliver both flavor and nutrients while meeting your dietary requirements following gastric sleeve surgery. From substantial chicken noodle soup to creamy tomato basil soup, each dish is intended to bring comfort and delight with each taste. Enjoy these easy yet savory soups as part of your post-surgery meal plan, ensuring that you get the nourishment you require while also indulging in wonderful flavors.

## Carrot and Ginger Soup

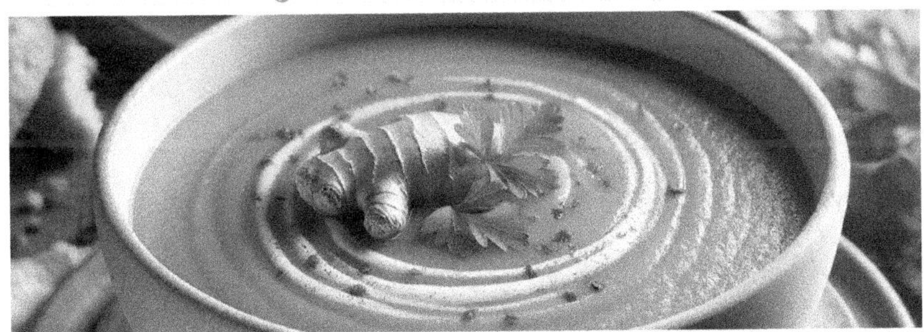

**Ingredients:**

- 4 cups carrots, peeled and chopped
- 1 onion, chopped
- 2 tablespoons fresh ginger, minced
- 4 cups vegetable broth
- 2 tablespoons olive oil
- Salt and pepper to taste

**Preparation:**

1. In a large pot, heat olive oil over medium heat.
2. Add chopped onions and ginger. Sauté for 3-4 minutes until fragrant.
3. Add chopped carrots and vegetable broth. Bring to a boil.
4. Reduce heat and simmer for 20-25 minutes, or until carrots are tender.
5. Use an immersion blender to puree the soup until smooth.
6. Season with salt and pepper to taste.
7. Serve hot.

**Cooking Time:** 30 minutes

**Nutritional Values** (approximate per serving):

- Calories: 120
- Protein: 2g
- Carbohydrates: 18g
- Fat: 5g
- Fiber: 4g
- Sugar: 8g

**Rating:** ★★★★☆

Carrot and Ginger Soup is a comforting and flavorful choice. The combination of sweet carrots and zesty ginger creates a delightful blend of flavors. This soup is not only easy to make but also provides essential nutrients while being gentle on your stomach. It's a perfect option for a light and nourishing meal, especially during your recovery period.

## Chicken Noodle Soup

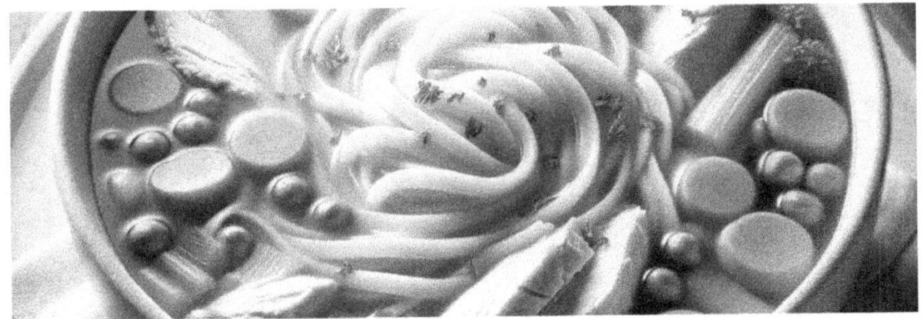

**Ingredients:**

- 2 boneless, skinless chicken breasts, cooked and shredded
- 4 cups low-sodium chicken broth
- 2 cups egg noodles
- 1 cup carrots, sliced
- 1 cup celery, chopped
- Salt and pepper to taste

**Preparation:**

1. In a large pot, bring chicken broth to a boil.
2. Add sliced carrots and chopped celery. Cook for 5-7 minutes until tender.

3. Add egg noodles and cook for another 7-8 minutes, or until noodles are tender.
4. Stir in the shredded chicken and cook until heated through.
5. Season with salt and pepper to taste.
6. Serve hot.

**Cooking Time:** 20 minutes

**Nutritional Values** (approximate per serving):

- Calories: 250
- Protein: 20g
- Carbohydrates: 25g
- Fat: 7g
- Fiber: 2g
- Sugar: 2g

**Rating:** ★★★★★

Chicken Noodle Soup is a classic and comforting choice. This soup combines tender chicken, hearty vegetables, and egg noodles in a flavorful chicken broth. It's not only delicious but also provides protein and essential nutrients. Whether enjoyed as a soothing meal during recovery or as a comforting dish on a chilly day, this soup is a go-to option for a satisfying and nourishing experience.

## Tomato Basil Soup

**Ingredients:**

- 4 cups canned tomato soup (low-sodium)
- 1 cup fresh basil leaves
- 1/2 cup heavy cream

- 1/4 cup grated Parmesan cheese
- Salt and pepper to taste

## Preparation:

1. In a blender, combine canned tomato soup and fresh basil leaves. Blend until smooth.
2. Pour the tomato basil mixture into a pot and heat over medium heat.
3. Stir in heavy cream and grated Parmesan cheese.
4. Cook for 5-7 minutes until heated through.
5. Season with salt and pepper to taste.
6. Serve hot.

**Cooking Time:** 10 minutes

**Nutritional Values** (approximate per serving):

- Calories: 200
- Protein: 4g
- Carbohydrates: 18g
- Fat: 13g
- Fiber: 2g
- Sugar: 8g

**Rating:** ★★★★☆

Tomato Basil Soup is a creamy and comforting choice. The combination of tangy tomato and aromatic basil creates a delightful flavor profile. This soup is quick to prepare and offers a rich and satisfying taste. It's a great option for a cozy and indulgent meal, perfect for those times when you crave a comforting and classic soup.

## Lentil Soup

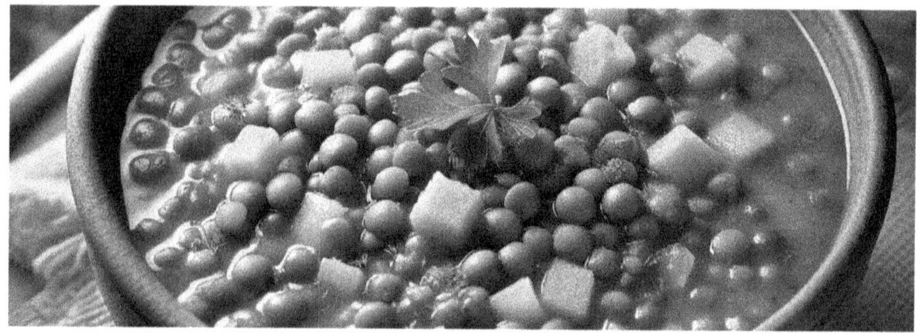

**Ingredients:**

- 1 cup dried green or brown lentils
- 4 cups vegetable broth
- 1 onion, chopped
- 2 carrots, chopped
- 2 celery stalks, chopped
- Salt and pepper to taste

**Preparation:**

1. Rinse lentils thoroughly and drain.
2. In a large pot, sauté chopped onions, carrots, and celery over medium heat until softened.

3. Add lentils and vegetable broth to the pot.

4. Bring to a boil, then reduce heat to a simmer and cook for 25-30 minutes, or until lentils are tender.

5. Season with salt and pepper to taste.

6. Serve hot.

**Cooking Time:** 35 minutes

**Nutritional Values** (approximate per serving):

- Calories: 200
- Protein: 13g
- Carbohydrates: 36g
- Fat: 1g
- Fiber: 10g
- Sugar: 5g

**Rating:** ★★★★☆

Lentil Soup is a hearty and nutritious option. Packed with protein and fiber, this soup is both filling and satisfying. The combination of lentils, vegetables, and vegetable broth creates a comforting and wholesome flavor. It's a simple yet nourishing choice for a balanced meal, making it an excellent addition to your bariatric diet.

## Pea and Ham Soup

**Ingredients:**

- 2 cups split green peas
- 1 cup ham, diced
- 1 onion, chopped
- 4 cups water
- Salt and pepper to taste

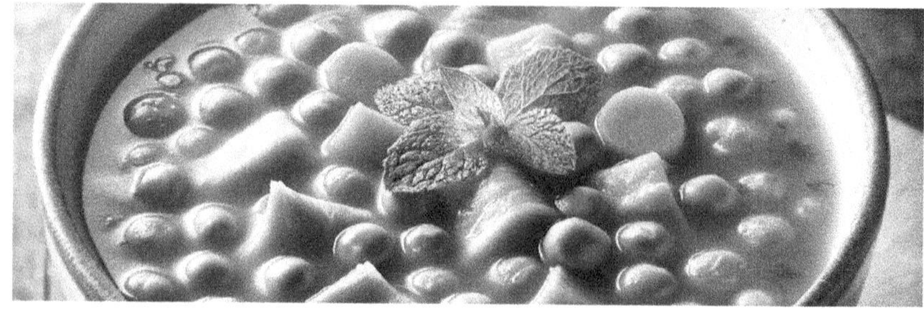

## Preparation:

1. Rinse split green peas thoroughly and drain.
2. In a large pot, combine split green peas, diced ham, chopped onions, and water.
3. Bring to a boil, then reduce heat to a simmer.
4. Cook for 45-60 minutes, or until split green peas are soft and the soup thickens.
5. Season with salt and pepper to taste.
6. Serve hot.

**Cooking Time:** 1 hour

**Nutritional Values** (approximate per serving):

- Calories: 250
- Protein: 18g
- Carbohydrates: 42g
- Fat: 2g
- Fiber: 16g
- Sugar: 6g

**Rating:** ★★★★☆

Pea and Ham Soup is a hearty and comforting choice. The combination of split green peas and diced ham creates a flavorful and satisfying soup. It's a source of protein and fiber, making it a filling option for your bariatric diet.

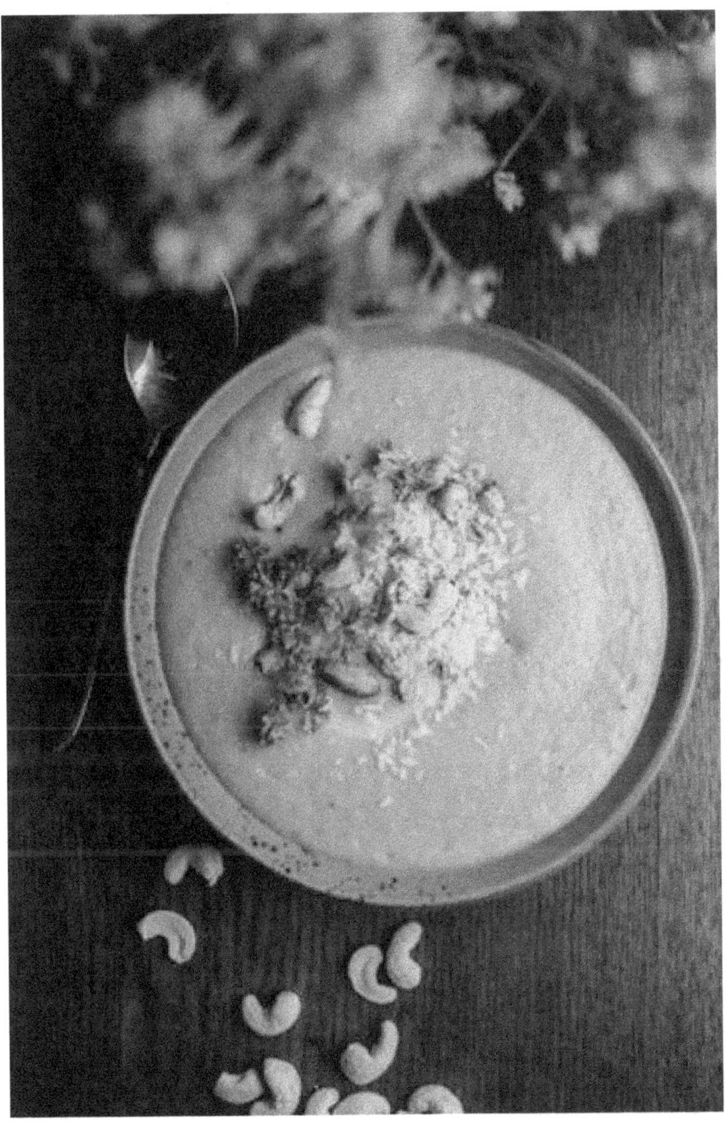

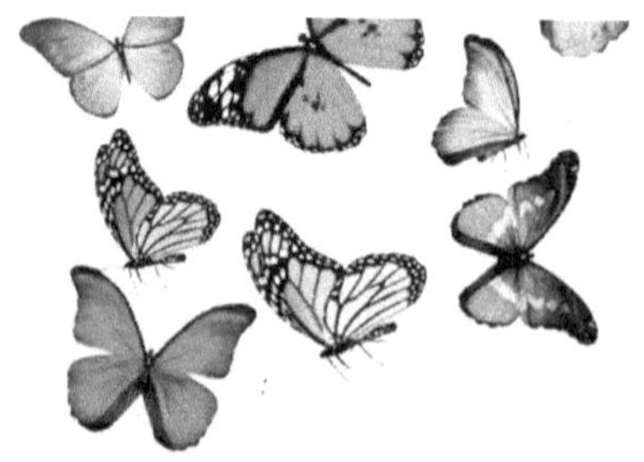

"Trust the process. Your journey with food post-gastric sleeve surgery is as much about transformation as it is about healing."

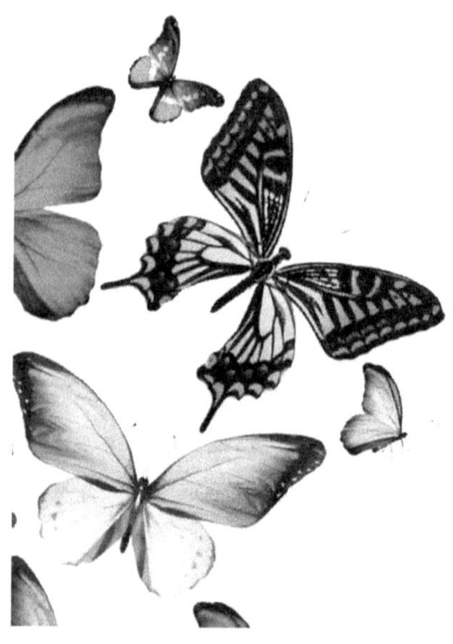

# Salads

Salads are a refreshing and nutritious supplement to your bariatric diet. Our salad recipes are intended to be easy, healthful, and full of flavor. With only five ingredients, these salads offer a range of textures and flavors to keep your meals interesting. From Spinach and Strawberry salad to Quinoa Tabbouleh, each recipe blends fresh vegetables with delectable sauces to create a filling and nutritious meal. These salads are an excellent way to get more veggies and protein into your diet while enjoying colorful tastes. These salads, whether as a side dish or a major entrée, are a tasty and healthy addition to your post-surgery diet.

## Spinach and Strawberry Salad

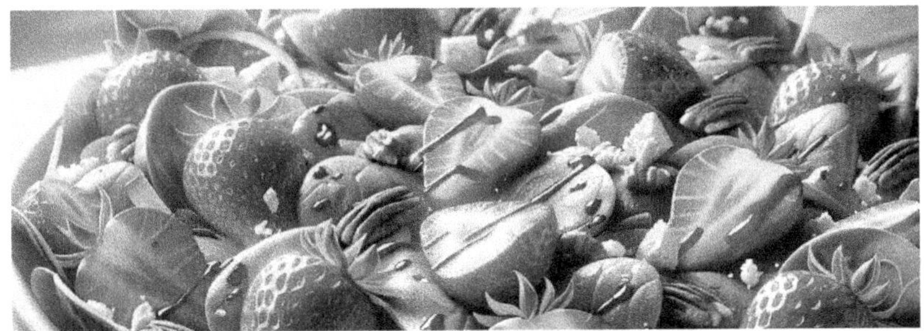

**Ingredients:**

- 4 cups fresh spinach leaves
- 1 cup strawberries, sliced
- 1/4 cup almonds, sliced and toasted
- 2 tablespoons balsamic vinaigrette dressing
- 1/4 cup feta cheese, crumbled

**Preparation:**

1. In a large bowl, combine fresh spinach leaves and sliced strawberries.
2. Drizzle balsamic vinaigrette dressing over the salad and toss to coat.
3. Top the salad with toasted almonds and crumbled feta cheese.
4. Serve immediately.

**Cooking Time:** No cooking required; preparation time is about 10 minutes.

**Nutritional Values** (approximate per serving):

- Calories: 150
- Protein: 4g
- Carbohydrates: 10g
- Fat: 11g
- Fiber: 3g
- Sugar: 5g

**Rating: ★★★★★**

Spinach and Strawberry Salad is a refreshing and delightful choice. The combination of fresh spinach, sweet strawberries, and the tangy balsamic vinaigrette creates a harmonious balance of flavors. Toasted almonds and crumbled feta cheese add a satisfying crunch and creaminess to the salad. It's a quick and nutritious option for a light and enjoyable meal.

## Cucumber, Tomato, and Feta Salad

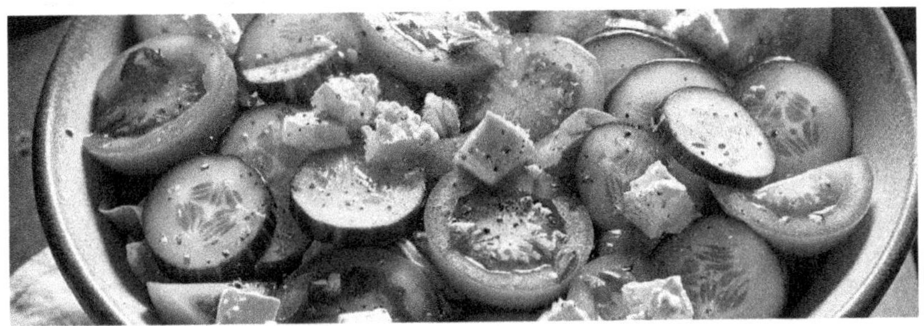

**Ingredients:**

- 2 cucumbers, diced
- 2 tomatoes, diced
- 1/2 cup feta cheese, crumbled
- 2 tablespoons olive oil
- 1 tablespoon red wine vinegar
- Fresh basil leaves for garnish (optional)

**Preparation:**

1. In a large bowl, combine diced cucumbers and tomatoes.
2. In a small bowl, whisk together olive oil and red wine vinegar to create the dressing.
3. Drizzle the dressing over the cucumber and tomato mixture.
4. Toss the salad to coat evenly.

5. Top with crumbled feta cheese and garnish with fresh basil leaves if desired.

6. Serve immediately.

**Cooking Time:** No cooking required; preparation time is about 10 minutes.

**Nutritional Values** (approximate per serving):

- Calories: 150
- Protein: 5g
- Carbohydrates: 8g
- Fat: 11g
- Fiber: 2g
- Sugar: 4g

**Rating:** ★★★★★

Cucumber, Tomato, and Feta Salad is a light and flavorful choice. The combination of crisp cucumbers, juicy tomatoes, and creamy feta cheese is complemented by the zesty dressing. It's a quick and healthy option for a refreshing side dish or a light meal. Enjoy the vibrant colors and delicious taste of this classic salad.

## Chicken Taco Salad

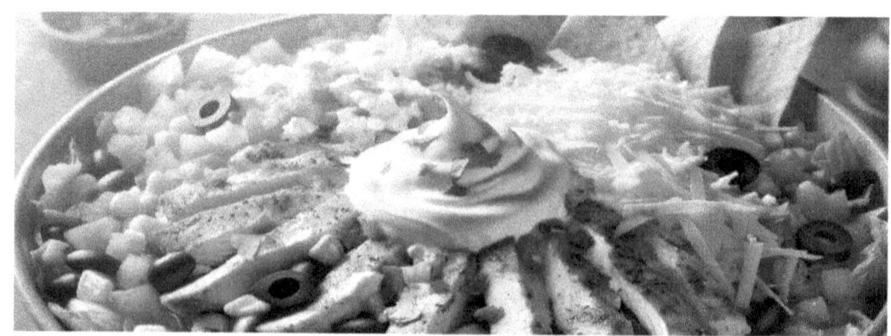

## Ingredients:

- 2 cups cooked chicken breast, shredded
- 4 cups romaine lettuce, chopped
- 1 cup cherry tomatoes, halved
- 1/4 cup cheddar cheese, shredded
- 2 tablespoons ranch dressing

## Preparation:

1. In a large bowl, combine chopped romaine lettuce, shredded chicken, cherry tomatoes, and cheddar cheese.
2. Drizzle ranch dressing over the salad and toss to coat.
3. Serve immediately.

**Cooking Time:** No cooking required; preparation time is about 10 minutes.

**Nutritional Values** (approximate per serving):

- Calories: 350
- Protein: 35g
- Carbohydrates: 10g
- Fat: 18g
- Fiber: 3g
- Sugar: 3g

**Rating:** ★★★★☆

This simplified Chicken Taco Salad recipe still delivers great taste with only 5 ingredients. Enjoy the delicious combination of shredded chicken, fresh romaine lettuce, cherry tomatoes, cheddar cheese, and ranch dressing for a quick and satisfying meal.

## Roasted Beet and Goat Cheese Salad

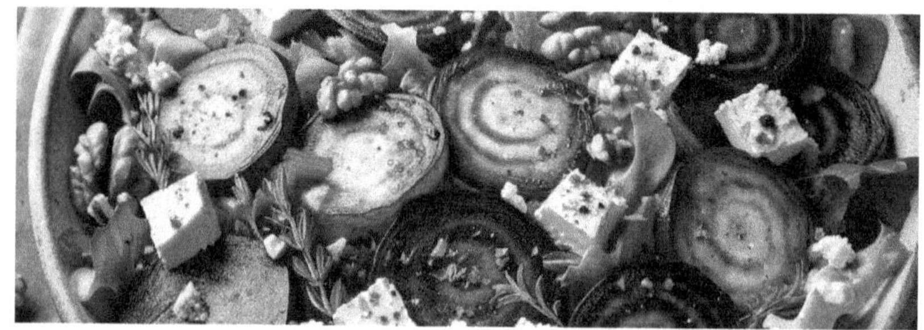

**Ingredients:**

- 4 medium-sized beets, roasted and sliced
- 2 cups mixed greens (e.g., arugula, spinach)
- 1/4 cup goat cheese, crumbled
- 2 tablespoons balsamic vinaigrette dressing
- 1/4 cup walnuts, chopped and toasted

**Preparation:**

1. Roast the beets: Preheat the oven to 400°F (200°C). Wrap the beets in foil and roast for about 45-60 minutes, or until tender. Let them cool, then peel and slice.
2. In a large bowl, combine the mixed greens and roasted beet slices.

3.  Drizzle balsamic vinaigrette dressing over the salad and toss to coat.

4.  Top with crumbled goat cheese and toasted walnuts.

5.  Serve immediately.

**Cooking Time:** Approximately 45-60 minutes for roasting the beets; no cooking required for the salad assembly.

**Nutritional Values** (approximate per serving):

- Calories: 200
- Protein: 6g
- Carbohydrates: 15g
- Fat: 14g
- Fiber: 4g
- Sugar: 10g

**Rating:** ★★★★★

Roasted Beet and Goat Cheese Salad is a vibrant and flavorful choice. The earthy sweetness of roasted beets combines perfectly with creamy goat cheese and toasted walnuts. The balsamic vinaigrette dressing adds a delightful tang. This salad is not only visually appealing but also rich in taste and texture, making it a wonderful option for a nutritious and delicious meal.

## Quinoa Tabbouleh

**Ingredients:**

- 1 cup quinoa, cooked and cooled
- 1 cup fresh parsley, chopped

- 1/2 cup cherry tomatoes, diced
- 1/4 cup red onion, finely chopped
- 2 tablespoons lemon juice
- Salt and pepper to taste

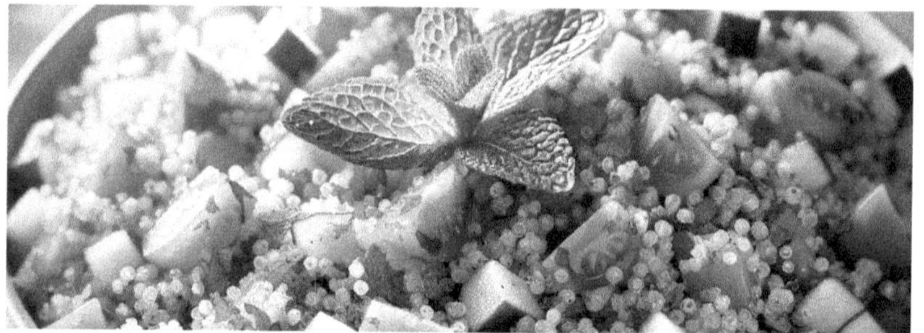

**Preparation:**

1. Cook quinoa according to package instructions and let it cool.
2. In a large bowl, combine cooked quinoa, chopped fresh parsley, diced cherry tomatoes, and finely chopped red onion.
3. Drizzle lemon juice over the mixture and toss to combine.
4. Season with salt and pepper to taste.
5. Serve chilled.

**Cooking Time:** Approximately 15-20 minutes to cook quinoa; preparation time is about 10 minutes.

**Nutritional Values** (approximate per serving):

- Calories: 200
- Protein: 5g
- Carbohydrates: 35g
- Fat: 4g
- Fiber: 5g
- Sugar: 2g

**Rating: ★★★★☆**

Quinoa Tabbouleh is a light and nutritious choice. This salad combines fluffy quinoa with fresh parsley, cherry tomatoes, and red onion, all tossed in a zesty lemon dressing. It's a refreshing and satisfying option for a quick and healthy meal. Enjoy the vibrant flavors and textures of this Mediterranean-inspired dish.

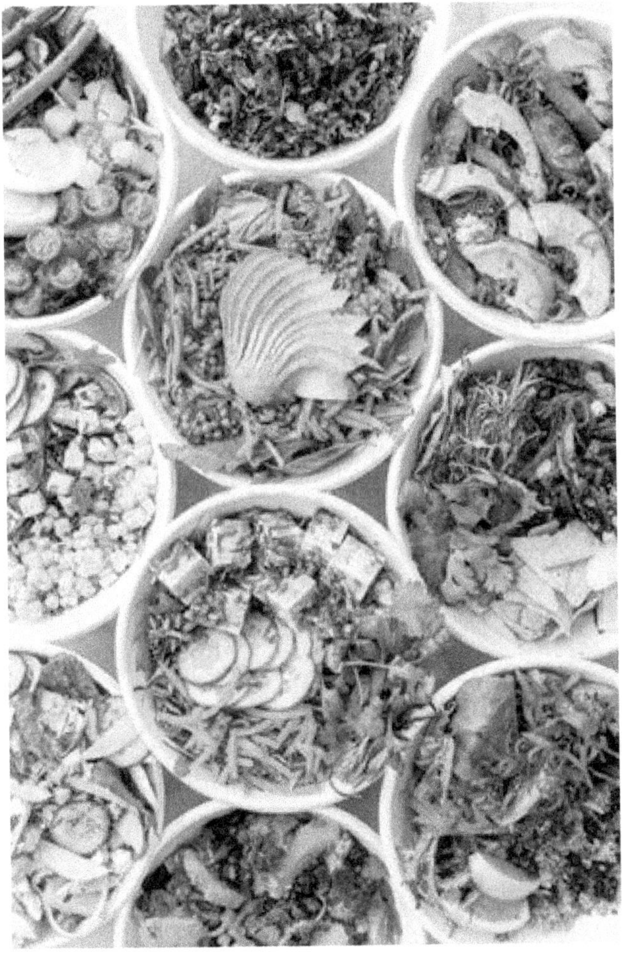

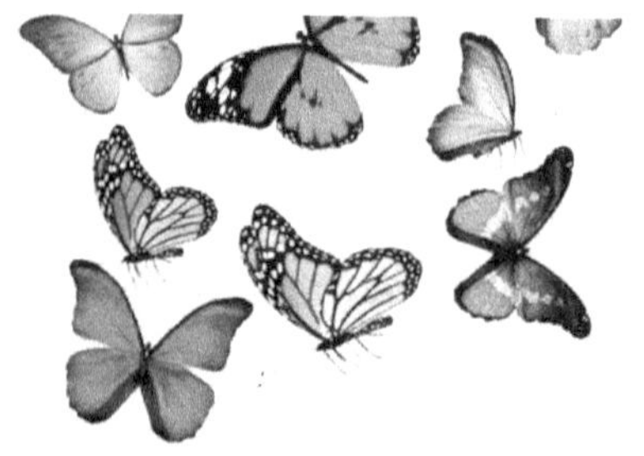

"Stay motivated by setting small, achievable goals. Each goal met is a stepping stone towards a healthier you."

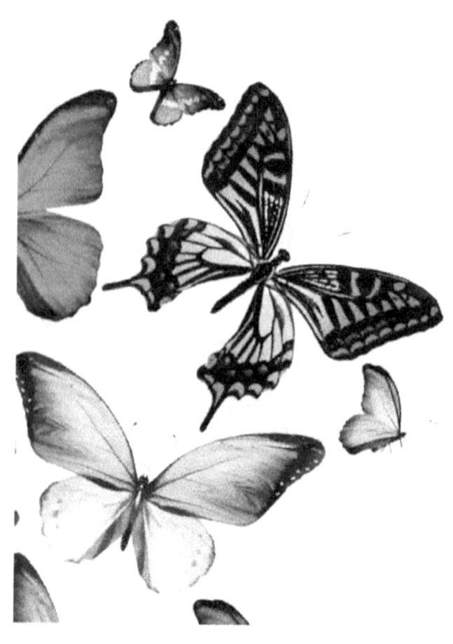

# Fish and Seafood

Fish and seafood offer a wonderful variety of flavors and textures for your bariatric diet. Our recipes are designed to be simple yet delicious, with just five ingredients in each dish. You'll find a range of options to satisfy your seafood cravings while meeting your dietary needs. These recipes are not only easy to prepare but also provide essential nutrients and healthy fats. Whether you prefer fish or seafood, these dishes are a tasty and nutritious addition to your post-surgery meal plan.

## Garlic Lemon Shrimp Skewers

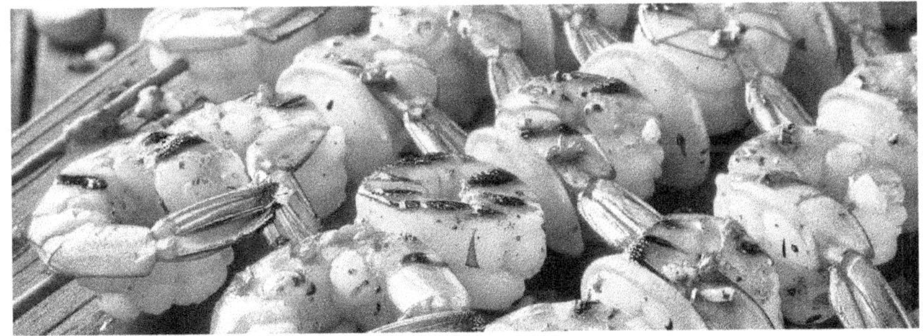

**Ingredients:**

- 1-pound large shrimp, peeled and deveined
- 2 cloves garlic, minced
- 2 tablespoons lemon juice
- 2 tablespoons olive oil
- Fresh parsley for garnish (optional)

**Preparation:**

1. In a bowl, combine minced garlic, lemon juice, and olive oil to create the marinade.
2. Thread the peeled and deveined shrimp onto skewers.
3. Brush the shrimp with the marinade on both sides.
4. Preheat a grill or grill pan to medium-high heat.
5. Grill the shrimp skewers for 2-3 minutes per side, or until they turn pink and opaque.
6. Garnish with fresh parsley if desired.
7. Serve hot.

**Cooking Time:** 5-6 minutes

**Nutritional Values** (approximate per serving):

- Calories: 150
- Protein: 20g
- Carbohydrates: 2g
- Fat: 7g
- Fiber: 0g
- Sugar: 0g

**Rating:** ★★★★☆

Garlic Lemon Shrimp Skewers are a quick and flavorful seafood option. The combination of garlic and lemon adds zesty and aromatic notes to the grilled shrimp. This dish is not only easy to prepare but also rich in protein, making it a satisfying choice for a seafood lover. Enjoy the succulent taste of these skewers as a delightful meal or a tasty appetizer.

## Baked Cod with Tomato and Basil

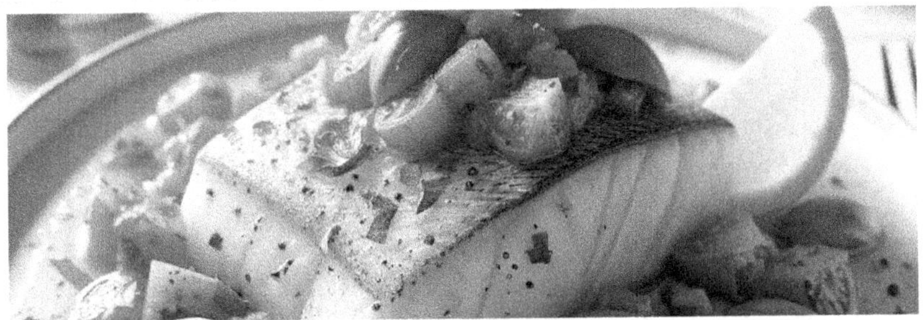

### Ingredients:

- 4 cod fillets
- 1 cup cherry tomatoes, halved
- 1/4 cup fresh basil leaves, chopped
- 2 tablespoons olive oil
- Salt and pepper to taste

### Preparation:

1. Preheat the oven to 375°F (190°C).
2. Place cod fillets in a baking dish.
3. In a bowl, combine cherry tomatoes, chopped fresh basil, olive oil, salt, and pepper.

4. Spoon the tomato and basil mixture over the cod fillets.

5. Cover the baking dish with foil.

6. Bake for 15-20 minutes, or until the cod flakes easily with a fork.

7. Serve hot.

**Cooking Time:** 15-20 minutes

**Nutritional Values** (approximate per serving):

- Calories: 200
- Protein: 25g
- Carbohydrates: 3g

- Fat: 9g
- Fiber: 1g
- Sugar: 1g

**Rating:** ★★★★☆

Baked Cod with Tomato and Basil is a light and flavorful seafood dish. The combination of juicy cherry tomatoes and fresh basil complements the mild taste of cod. Baking the cod in this tomato and basil mixture infuses it with delicious flavors.

## Pan-Seared Scallops with Quinoa

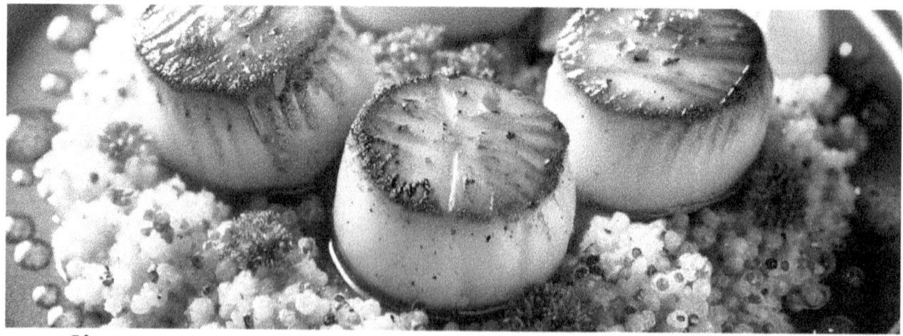

**Ingredients:**

- 1 pound sea scallops
- 1 cup quinoa, cooked
- 2 tablespoons olive oil
- 2 cloves garlic, minced
- Fresh lemon wedges for garnish (optional)

**Preparation:**

1. Pat dry the scallops with a paper towel to remove excess moisture.
2. Heat olive oil in a skillet over medium-high heat.
3. Add minced garlic and sauté for about 30 seconds.
4. Add the scallops to the skillet and sear for 2-3 minutes per side, or until they develop a golden crust and are opaque in the center.
5. Serve the scallops over cooked quinoa.
6. Garnish with fresh lemon wedges if desired.
7. Serve hot.

**Cooking Time:** 5-6 minutes

**Nutritional Values** (approximate per serving):

- Calories: 300
- Protein: 25g
- Carbohydrates: 25g
- Fat: 10g
- Fiber: 3g
- Sugar: 0g

**Rating:** ★★★★☆

Pan-Seared Scallops with Quinoa is a delightful seafood dish. The scallops are seared to perfection, creating a beautiful crust while remaining tender on the inside. Served over fluffy quinoa, it's a protein-rich and satisfying meal. The addition of garlic and optional lemon wedges adds flavor and zest to this elegant dish, making it a great choice for a special occasion or a delicious weeknight dinner.

## Salmon Patties

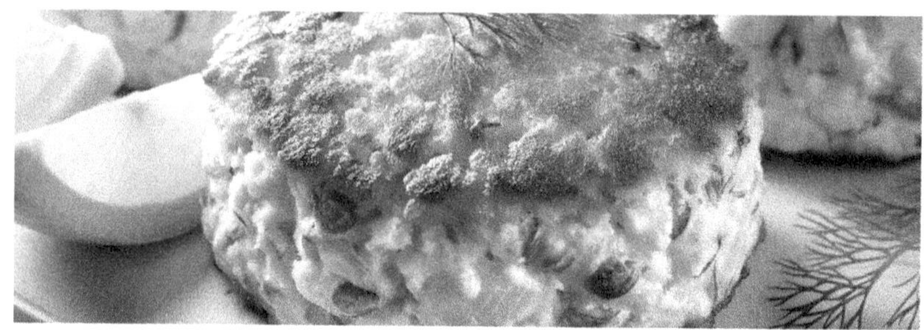

**Ingredients:**

- 2 cans (14 ounces each) canned salmon, drained and flaked
- 1/2 cup breadcrumbs
- 1/4 cup mayonnaise
- 1 egg
- 1/4 cup chopped fresh parsley
- Lemon wedges for serving (optional)

**Preparation:**

1. In a bowl, combine canned salmon, breadcrumbs, mayonnaise, egg, and chopped fresh parsley.
2. Mix until well combined.
3. Form the mixture into patties.
4. Heat a skillet over medium-high heat and lightly grease it.

5. Cook the salmon patties for 3-4 minutes per side, or until they are golden brown and heated through.

6. Serve with lemon wedges if desired.

**Cooking Time:** 8-10 minutes

**Nutritional Values** (approximate per serving, without lemon wedges):

- Calories: 200
- Protein: 20g
- Carbohydrates: 8g
- Fat: 10g
- Fiber: 1g
- Sugar: 1g

**Rating:** ★★★★☆

Salmon Patties are a flavorful and protein-packed seafood choice. These patties are made with canned salmon, breadcrumbs, and seasonings, creating a crispy exterior and a tender interior. They are quick to prepare and make for a satisfying meal. Enjoy them with a squeeze of lemon for added zest and freshness

## Tilapia with Mango Salsa

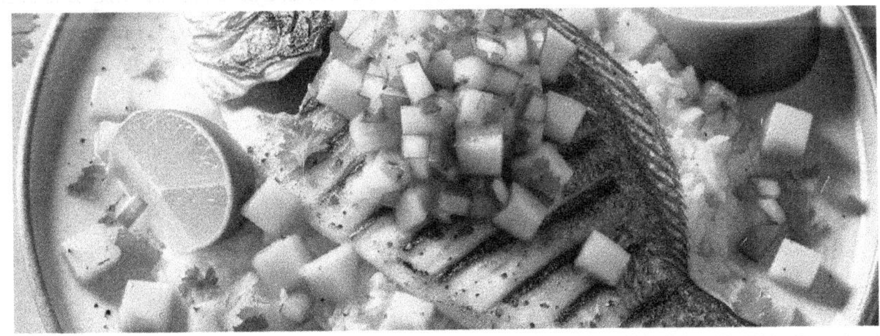

## Ingredients:

- 4 tilapia fillets
- 1 ripe mango, diced
- 1/4 cup red onion, finely chopped
- 1/4 cup fresh cilantro, chopped
- 2 tablespoons lime juice
- Salt and pepper to taste

## Preparation:

1. Season tilapia fillets with salt and pepper.

2. In a bowl, combine diced mango, finely chopped red onion, fresh cilantro, and lime juice to create the salsa.

3. Preheat a skillet over medium-high heat and lightly grease it.

4. Cook the tilapia fillets for 3-4 minutes per side, or until they are cooked through and flake easily with a fork.

5. Serve the tilapia topped with mango salsa.

**Cooking Time:** 6-8 minutes

**Nutritional Values** (approximate per serving):

- Calories: 200
- Protein: 25g
- Carbohydrates: 18g
- Fat: 2g
- Fiber: 2g
- Sugar: 14g

**Rating:** ★★★★☆

Tilapia with Mango Salsa is a light and tropical seafood dish. The tilapia fillets are seasoned and cooked to perfection, while the mango salsa adds a sweet and tangy flavor with a hint of freshness from cilantro. This combination makes for a delicious and visually appealing meal that's quick to prepare and perfect for your bariatric diet.

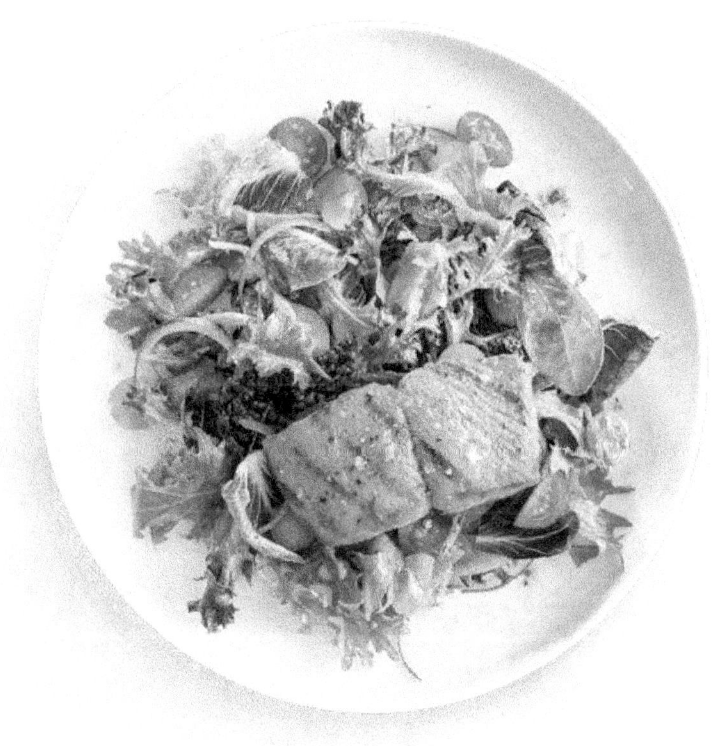

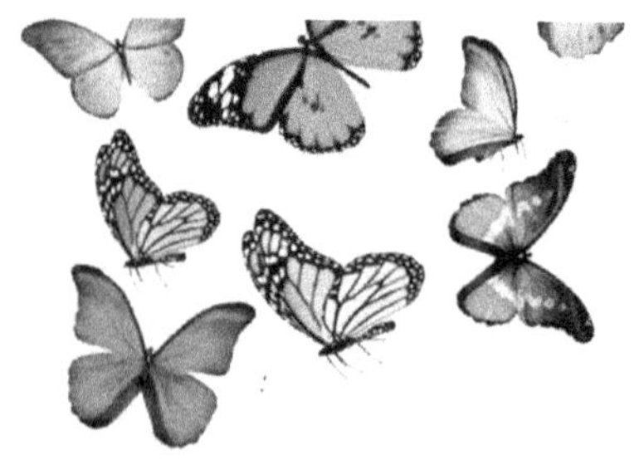

"Remember why you started. Your journey is unique and every healthy meal is a testament to your strength and dedication."

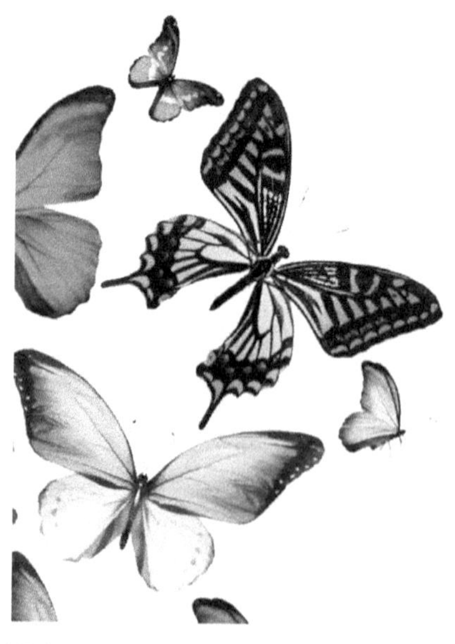

# Beverages

Beverages are a crucial component of any meal plan, and we offer some refreshing alternatives to supplement your bariatric diet. These beverages, which range from infused water concoctions to protein-packed smoothies, are intended to keep you hydrated while also providing necessary nutrients. Each recipe requires only five ingredients, making it simple to prepare and enjoy. Whether you're searching for a morning pick-me-up or a delightful post-workout drink, our beverage recipes come in a range of flavors to fit your taste while keeping your dietary requirements in mind.

## Berry Protein Smoothie

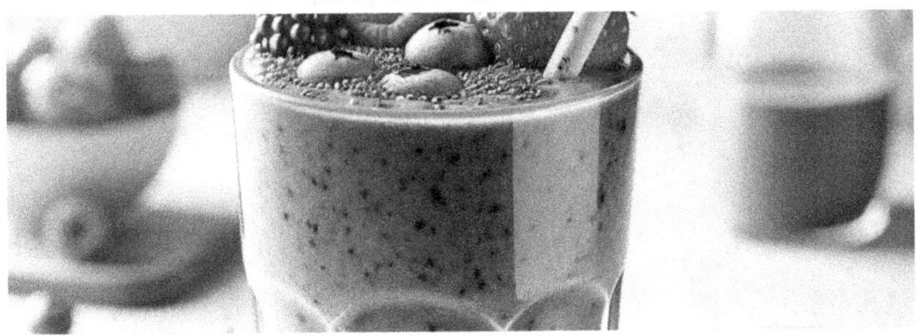

**Ingredients:**

- 1 cup mixed berries (e.g., strawberries, blueberries, raspberries)
- 1 cup Greek yogurt
- 1/2 cup unsweetened almond milk
- 1 scoop vanilla protein powder
- 1 tablespoon honey (optional for sweetness)

**Preparation:**

1. Place mixed berries, Greek yogurt, unsweetened almond milk, vanilla protein powder, and honey (if desired) in a blender.

2. Blend until smooth and creamy.

3. Serve chilled.

**Cooking Time:** No cooking required; preparation time is about 5 minutes.

**Nutritional Values** (approximate per serving, without honey):

- Calories: 250
- Protein: 25g
- Carbohydrates: 25g
- Fat: 5g
- Fiber: 5g
- Sugar: 15g

**Rating: ★★★★☆**

The Berry Protein Smoothie is a delicious and protein-packed beverage. It combines the goodness of mixed berries, Greek yogurt, and protein powder for a satisfying and nutritious drink. The honey adds a touch of sweetness, making it a delightful option for a quick and energizing snack or breakfast. Enjoy the refreshing flavors and the boost of protein with this smoothie.

## Cucumber Mint Water

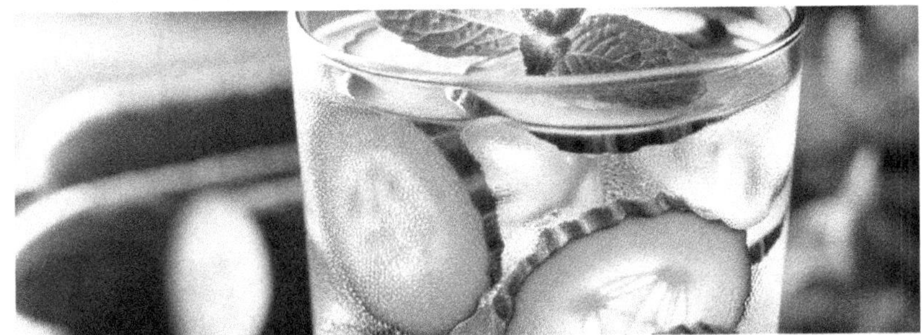

### Ingredients:

- 1 cucumber, thinly sliced
- 1/4 cup fresh mint leaves
- 8 cups water
- Ice cubes (optional)
- Lemon or lime slices (optional for extra flavor)

### Preparation:

1. Place cucumber slices and fresh mint leaves in a pitcher.
2. Add 8 cups of water to the pitcher.
3. Refrigerate for at least 2 hours to allow flavors to infuse.
4. Serve chilled, with ice cubes and lemon or lime slices if desired.

**Cooking Time:** No cooking required; infusing time is about 2 hours.

**Nutritional Values** (approximate per serving, without optional ingredients):

- Calories: 0
- Protein: 0g
- Carbohydrates: 0g
- Fat: 0g
- Fiber: 0g
- Sugar: 0g

**Rating: ★★★★☆**

Cucumber Mint Water is a refreshing and hydrating beverage. The combination of cucumber and fresh mint gives a cool and invigorating flavor to plain water. It's a great way to stay hydrated throughout the day, and you can customize it with ice cubes or citrus slices for extra freshness. Enjoy this simple and healthy drink as a thirst-quencher.

## Almond Milk Hot Cocoa

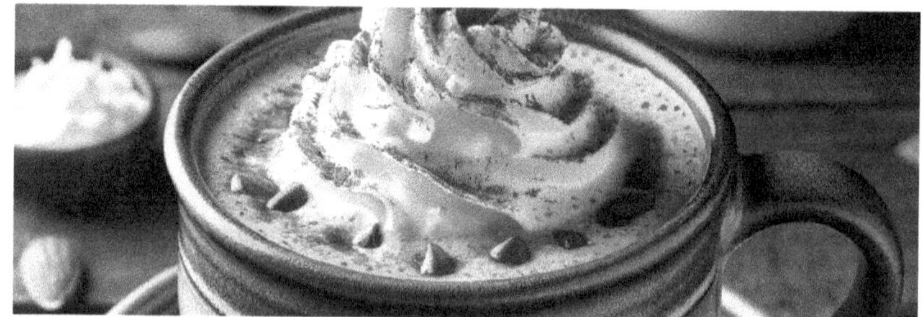

**Ingredients:**

- 2 cups unsweetened almond milk
- 2 tablespoons unsweetened cocoa powder
- 2 tablespoons honey or maple syrup (adjust to taste)
- 1/2 teaspoon vanilla extract

- Pinch of salt

**Preparation:**

1. In a saucepan, heat unsweetened almond milk over medium heat until warm (do not boil).
2. Whisk in unsweetened cocoa powder, honey or maple syrup, vanilla extract, and a pinch of salt.
3. Continue to whisk until the cocoa powder is fully dissolved and the mixture is smooth.
4. Pour the hot cocoa into mugs and serve.

**Cooking Time:** Approximately 5 minutes

**Nutritional Values** (approximate per serving, using honey):

- Calories: 80
- Protein: 1g
- Carbohydrates: 16g
- Fat: 2g
- Fiber: 2g
- Sugar: 12g

**Rating:** ★★★★☆

Almond Milk Hot Cocoa is a comforting and dairy-free beverage. It combines the richness of cocoa with the subtle sweetness of almond milk, making it a delightful treat for a cozy evening. Adjust the sweetness to your preference with honey or maple syrup. Enjoy the warm and chocolaty goodness of this hot cocoa without the need for dairy.

## Green Detox Juice

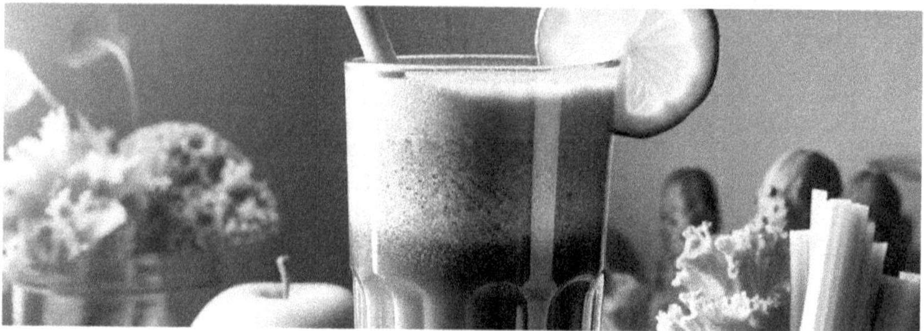

### Ingredients:

- 2 cups kale leaves, stems removed
- 2 green apples, cored and sliced
- 1 cucumber, peeled and sliced
- 1 lemon, peeled and sliced
- 1-inch piece of ginger, peeled

### Preparation:

1. Place kale leaves, green apples, cucumber, lemon slices, and ginger in a juicer.
2. Process all the ingredients through the juicer.
3. Stir the juice well to combine.
4. Serve immediately over ice if desired.

**Cooking Time:** No cooking required; juicing time is a few minutes.

**Nutritional Values** (approximate per serving):

- Calories: 120
- Protein: 2g

- Carbohydrates: 30g
- Fat: 1g
- Fiber: 6g
- Sugar: 15g

**Rating:** ★★★★☆

Green Detox Juice is a nutrient-packed and refreshing beverage. This green juice combines the cleansing power of kale, the natural sweetness of green apples, the hydrating qualities of cucumber, the zing of lemon, and the warmth of ginger. It's a great way to boost your energy and get essential vitamins and minerals. Enjoy this rejuvenating and healthful drink as part of your wellness routine.

## Herbal Tea Blends for Digestion

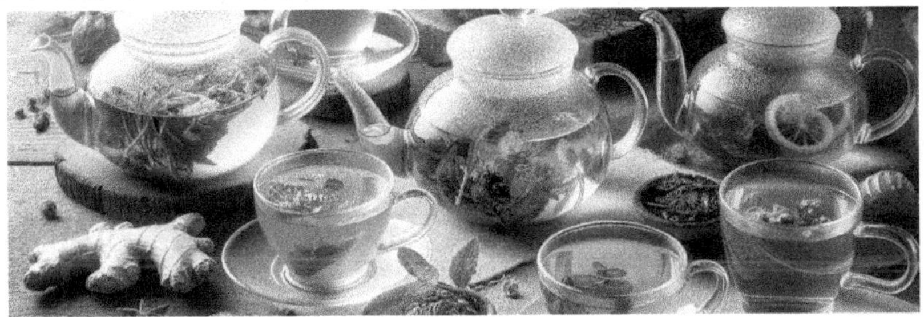

**Ingredients:**

- 1 teaspoon dried peppermint leaves
- 1 teaspoon dried ginger root
- 1 teaspoon fennel seeds
- 1 teaspoon chamomile flowers
- 8-10 ounces boiling water

**Preparation:**

1. Place dried peppermint leaves, dried ginger root, fennel seeds, and chamomile flowers in a tea infuser or a tea bag.
2. Pour boiling water over the herbs in a cup.
3. Cover and steep for 5-7 minutes.
4. Remove the tea infuser or bag.
5. Serve hot and enjoy.

**Cooking Time:** 5-7 minutes (steeping time)

**Nutritional Values** (approximate per serving):

- Calories: 0
- Protein: 0g
- Carbohydrates: 0g
- Fat: 0g
- Fiber: 0g
- Sugar: 0g

**Rating:** ★★★★☆

Herbal Tea Blends for Digestion is a soothing and aromatic tea that promotes digestive wellness. This herbal blend combines the digestive benefits of peppermint, ginger, fennel, and chamomile. It's a gentle and natural way to ease digestive discomfort and support overall gut health. Enjoy this tea after meals or anytime you need a calming and digestive-friendly beverage.

# Meal Planning and Strategies

Meal planning is your roadmap to success on your bariatric journey. It's about making smart choices, ensuring you get the right nutrients, and controlling portions. With meal planning, you can save time, minimize waste, and reduce stress. This guide will provide practical tips to make meal planning simple and effective for your health and weight goals.

## 7 Days Meal Plan Sample

**Day 1**

- **Breakfast:** Protein-Packed Greek Yogurt Parfait

- **Lunch:** Turkey and Avocado Roll-Ups

- **Dinner:** Baked Salmon with Asparagus

- **Snack:** Cucumber and Hummus Bites

- **Dessert:** Almond Butter Banana Cookies

**Day 2**

- **Breakfast:** Savory Egg Muffins

- **Lunch:** Chickpea Salad with Lemon Vinaigrette

- **Dinner:** Chicken and Broccoli Stir-Fry

- **Snack:** Greek Yogurt and Berry Compote

- **Dessert:** Ricotta and Berry Compote

**Day 3**

- **Breakfast:** Banana and Almond Smoothie Bowl

- **Lunch:** Cottage Cheese and Fruit Bowl

- **Dinner:** Zucchini Noodles with Tomato Sauce

- **Snack:** Avocado Chocolate Mousse

- **Dessert:** Baked Pear with Honey and Walnuts

**Day 4**

- **Breakfast:** Spinach and Feta Omelet Cups

- **Lunch:** Tuna Stuffed Bell Peppers

- **Dinner:** Turkey Meatball Soup

- **Snack:** Roasted Brussels Sprouts with Balsamic Glaze

- **Dessert:** Cocoa and Avocado Smoothie

**Day 5**

- **Breakfast:** Quinoa and Berry Breakfast Porridge

- **Lunch:** Quinoa Vegetable Soup

- **Dinner:** Cauliflower Fried Rice

- **Snack:** Cucumber and Dill Salad

- **Dessert:** Coconut Flour Pancakes

**Day 6**

- **Breakfast:** Lemon Herb Chicken Breast

- **Lunch:** Garlic Lime Pork Chops

- **Dinner:** Baked Cod with Lemon and Dill

- **Snack:** Mixed Bean Salad

- **Dessert:** Spinach and Strawberry Salad

**Day 7**

- **Breakfast:** Chicken and Broccoli Stir-Fry

- **Lunch:** Baked Turkey Meatballs

- **Dinner:** Seafood Stir-Fry

- **Snack:** Green Detox Smoothie

- **Dessert:** Mixed Bean Salad

Feel free to adjust portion sizes to meet your dietary needs and preferences. Enjoy your delicious and nutritious meals!

## Meal Planning and Prep for the Week

Meal planning and preparation for the week is a key strategy to help you stay on track with your bariatric diet and maintain a healthy eating routine. Here are some tips to make the process easier and more effective:

**1. Choose Your Recipes:** Start by selecting the recipes you want to prepare for the week. Refer to your meal plan and make a list of the dishes you'll be making.

**2. Make a Shopping List:** Based on your chosen recipes, create a detailed shopping list. Ensure you have all the ingredients you need to avoid last-minute grocery trips.

**3. Set Aside Dedicated Time:** Block out a specific time in your schedule for meal preparation. This can be on a weekend or a convenient day during the week.

**4. Prep Ingredients:** Before you start cooking, wash, chop, and prepare all the ingredients you'll need. This includes vegetables, meats, and any other components of your recipes.

**5. Cook in Batches:** Cook large batches of meals that can be divided into portions for the week. This can save you time and effort on busy days.

**6. Use Portion-Control Containers:** Invest in portion-control containers to divide your meals into appropriate serving sizes. This makes it easier to stick to your portion control goals.

**7. Label and Store:** Label your containers with the date and contents to keep track of freshness. Store meals in the refrigerator or freezer, depending on when you plan to consume them.

**8. Mix and Match:** Prepare versatile ingredients that can be used in various dishes throughout the week. For example, roasted vegetables can be added to salads, wraps, or served as sides.

**9. Plan for Snacks:** Don't forget to prep healthy snacks like cut fruits, yogurt, or nuts for those moments when you need a quick bite.

**10. Stay Organized:** Keep your kitchen organized with clear labeling, and arrange your meals in a way that makes it easy to grab what you need.

**11. Stay Consistent:** Try to stick to your meal plan as closely as possible throughout the week. Consistency is key to achieving your dietary goals.

**12. Be Flexible:** While planning is important, be flexible enough to adapt to changes in your schedule or cravings. Having healthy options readily available can help you make better choices.

By dedicating time to meal planning and preparation, you'll set yourself up for success on your bariatric journey. It reduces the temptation to make unhealthy food choices and ensures that you have nutritious meals at your fingertips, making it easier to achieve your weight loss and health goals.

## Shopping Tips for Simple, Healthy Ingredients

Shopping for simple, healthy ingredients is a crucial part of maintaining a balanced bariatric diet. Here are some shopping tips to help you make nutritious choices at the grocery store:

**1. Plan Your Meals:** Before heading to the store, create a meal plan for the week. Knowing what you need will prevent you from making impulsive purchases.

**2. Make a List:** Based on your meal plan, make a detailed shopping list. Organize it by sections like produce, proteins, dairy, etc., to navigate the store efficiently.

**3. Shop the Perimeter:** In most grocery stores, fresh and unprocessed foods like fruits, vegetables, lean proteins, and dairy are located around the perimeter. Focus on these areas for healthier options.

**4. Read Labels:** When buying packaged foods, read the nutrition labels carefully. Look for products with lower sugar, saturated fat, and sodium content.

**5. Choose Whole Grains:** Opt for whole grains like brown rice, quinoa, and whole wheat bread over refined grains. They are higher in fiber and more nutritious.

**6. Prioritize Lean Proteins:** Select lean cuts of meat like skinless poultry, lean beef, and fish. Consider plant-based protein sources like tofu and legumes.

**7. Buy Fresh Produce:** Fresh fruits and vegetables are rich in vitamins and minerals. Choose a variety of colorful options to ensure you get a wide range of nutrients.

**8. Minimize Processed Foods:** Reduce your intake of processed and pre-packaged foods, which often contain additives, preservatives, and excess salt and sugar.

**9. Stock up on Healthy Snacks:** Purchase healthy snacks like Greek yogurt, nuts, and cut-up vegetables to have on hand for quick, satisfying snacks.

**10. Avoid Sugary Drinks:** Limit sugary beverages like soda and fruit juices. Opt for water, herbal tea, or sparkling water instead.

**11. Check for Sales and Discounts:** Take advantage of sales and discounts to save money on healthy items. Buying in bulk can also be cost-effective.

**12. Be Mindful of Portion Sizes:** Pay attention to portion sizes when buying items like nuts or dried fruits. It's easy to overconsume these calorie-dense foods.

**13. Don't Shop Hungry:** Avoid shopping when you're hungry, as it can lead to impulse purchases of unhealthy snacks.

**14. Consider Frozen and Canned Options:** Frozen fruits and vegetables can be just as nutritious as fresh ones and have a longer shelf life. Canned options like beans and tomatoes are convenient for recipes.

**15. Embrace Variety:** Keep your diet interesting by trying new foods and ingredients regularly. Experimenting with different flavors and cuisines can make healthy eating enjoyable.

By following these shopping tips and making informed choices, you can fill your pantry and refrigerator with simple, healthy ingredients that support your bariatric journey and overall well-being.

## Essential Ingredients list

**1. Lean Proteins:**

- Skinless chicken breasts
- Lean ground turkey or chicken
- Salmon or other fatty fish
- Lean cuts of beef or pork
- Tofu or tempeh (for vegetarians)

**2. Fruits:**

- Apples
- Berries (strawberries, blueberries, etc.)
- Bananas
- Citrus fruits (oranges, lemons, etc.)
- Avocado

## 3. Vegetables:

- Leafy greens (spinach, kale, lettuce)
- Broccoli
- Cauliflower
- Bell peppers
- Zucchini

## 4. Whole Grains:

- Quinoa
- Brown rice
- Whole wheat pasta
- Oats
- Whole grain bread

## 5. Legumes:

- Black beans
- Chickpeas
- Lentils
- Kidney beans
- Pinto beans

## 6. Dairy and Dairy Alternatives:

- Greek yogurt (low-fat or non-fat)
- Low-fat or almond milk
- Low-fat cheese (if tolerated)

## 7. Nuts and Seeds:

- Almonds
- Walnuts

- Chia seeds
- Flaxseeds

## 8. Herbs and Spices:

- Garlic
- Oregano
- Onion
- Cumin
- Basil

## 9. Healthy Fats:

- Olive oil
- Avocado oil
- Coconut oil

**10. Condiments and Sauces:** - Low-sodium soy sauce - Mustard - Vinegar (balsamic, apple cider) - Hot sauce (if tolerated)

**11. Sweeteners:** - Honey - Maple syrup - Stevia (in moderation)

**12. Frozen and Canned Foods:** - Frozen fruits and vegetables - Canned tomatoes - Frozen lean protein options (e.g., fish fillets)

**13. Baking Essentials (if applicable):** - Whole wheat flour - Baking powder - Baking soda

**14. Beverages:** - Water (hydration is key) - Herbal tea - Sugar-free or low-sugar beverages

**15. Supplements (as advised by your healthcare provider):** - Multivitamins - Calcium supplements - Vitamin B12 (if required)

**16. Fresh Herbs:** - Parsley - Cilantro - Mint

Having these essential ingredients on hand will make it easier to prepare nutritious and delicious meals while following your bariatric dietary guidelines. Adjust the list to suit your specific dietary preferences and consult with your healthcare provider for personalized recommendations.

## Managing Portion Sizes and Nutritional Intake

Here are some tips to help you effectively manage your portions and ensure you're getting the right nutrients:

**1. Use Smaller Plates:** Opt for smaller plates and bowls to help control portion sizes. This can trick your brain into thinking you're eating more.

**2. Measure Your Food:** Invest in measuring cups and a kitchen scale to accurately measure your portions, especially for proteins, grains, and snacks.

**3. Follow Your Healthcare Provider's Recommendations:** Your healthcare team will provide guidelines on portion sizes based on your specific surgery and needs. Follow their recommendations closely.

**4. Focus on Protein:** Prioritize protein-rich foods in your meals as they promote satiety and muscle preservation. Aim for lean sources like chicken, fish, tofu, and beans.

**5. Fill Half Your Plate with Vegetables:** Load up on non-starchy vegetables like leafy greens, broccoli, and peppers. They are low in calories and high in nutrients.

**6. Avoid Grazing:** Stick to planned meals and snacks, and avoid grazing throughout the day. This can help prevent overeating.

**7. Practice Mindful Eating:** Pay attention to hunger and fullness cues. Eat slowly, savor each bite, and stop when you're comfortably satisfied, not overly full.

**8. Stay Hydrated:** Drink water throughout the day to stay hydrated. Sometimes thirst can be mistaken for hunger.

**9. Plan Balanced Meals:** Include a balance of protein, vegetables, and whole grains in your meals to ensure you're getting a variety of nutrients.

**10. Limit Liquid Calories:** Be cautious with high-calorie beverages like sugary drinks and alcohol, as they can add unnecessary calories.

**11. Avoid High-Calorie Snacking:** Opt for healthy snacks like fruits, Greek yogurt, or nuts instead of calorie-dense snacks.

**12. Keep a Food Diary:** Tracking your food intake can help you become more aware of your eating habits and make adjustments as needed.

**13. Avoid Emotional Eating:** Find alternative ways to cope with stress or emotions rather than turning to food for comfort.

**14. Follow Dietary Guidelines:** Adhere to your healthcare provider's dietary guidelines, including recommendations for vitamins and supplements.

**15. Consult a Dietitian:** Consider working with a registered dietitian who specializes in bariatric nutrition. They can provide personalized guidance and support.

**16. Be Patient:** Weight loss may not always be linear, and plateaus are common. Stay consistent with your healthy eating habits and exercise patience.

Remember that managing portion sizes and nutritional intake is an ongoing process. It's important to develop a healthy relationship with food and make sustainable lifestyle changes to support your long-term health and weight loss goals.

For further Questions and advice reach out on

joanmilonehelpdesk@gmail.com

# Thank You

I'm writing this with a heart full of gratitude for your kind words and the time you took to read my book, knowing that my words have resonated with you is a reward beyond measure. Thank you again for your appreciation and for being a part of this literary journey.

Warmly,

*Joan*

# 30 Days Meal Planner

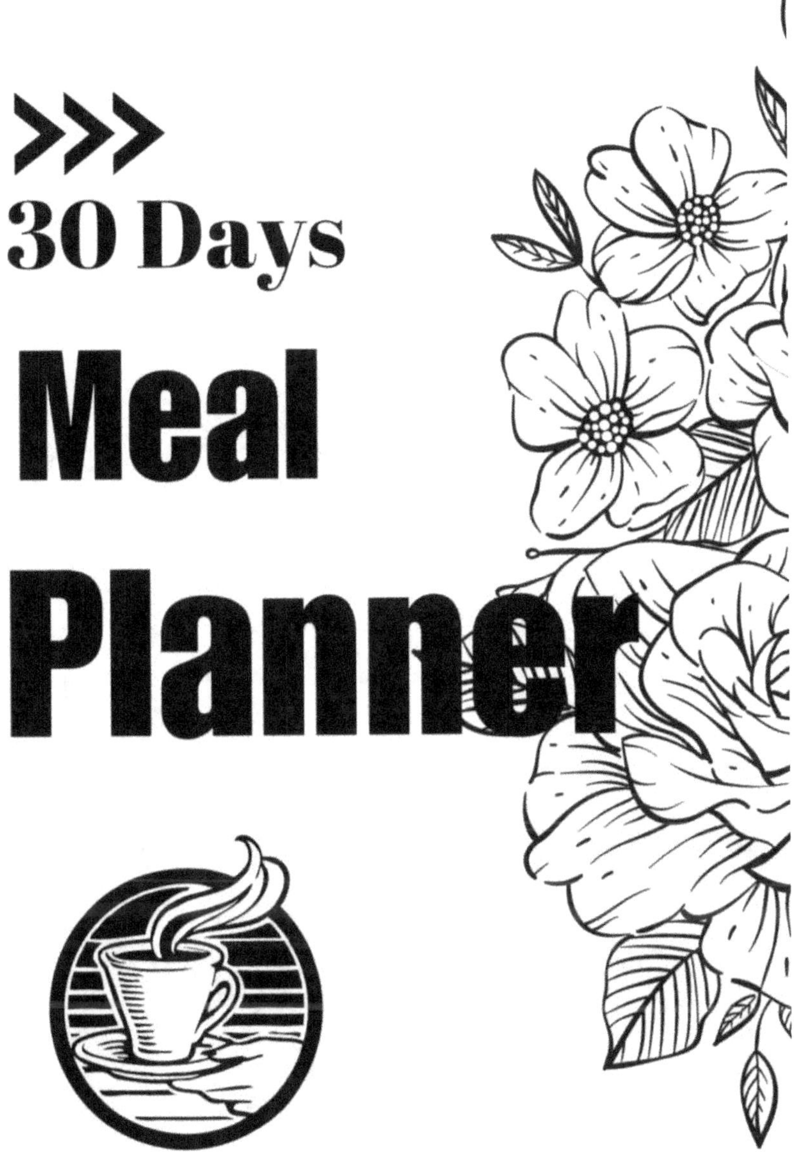

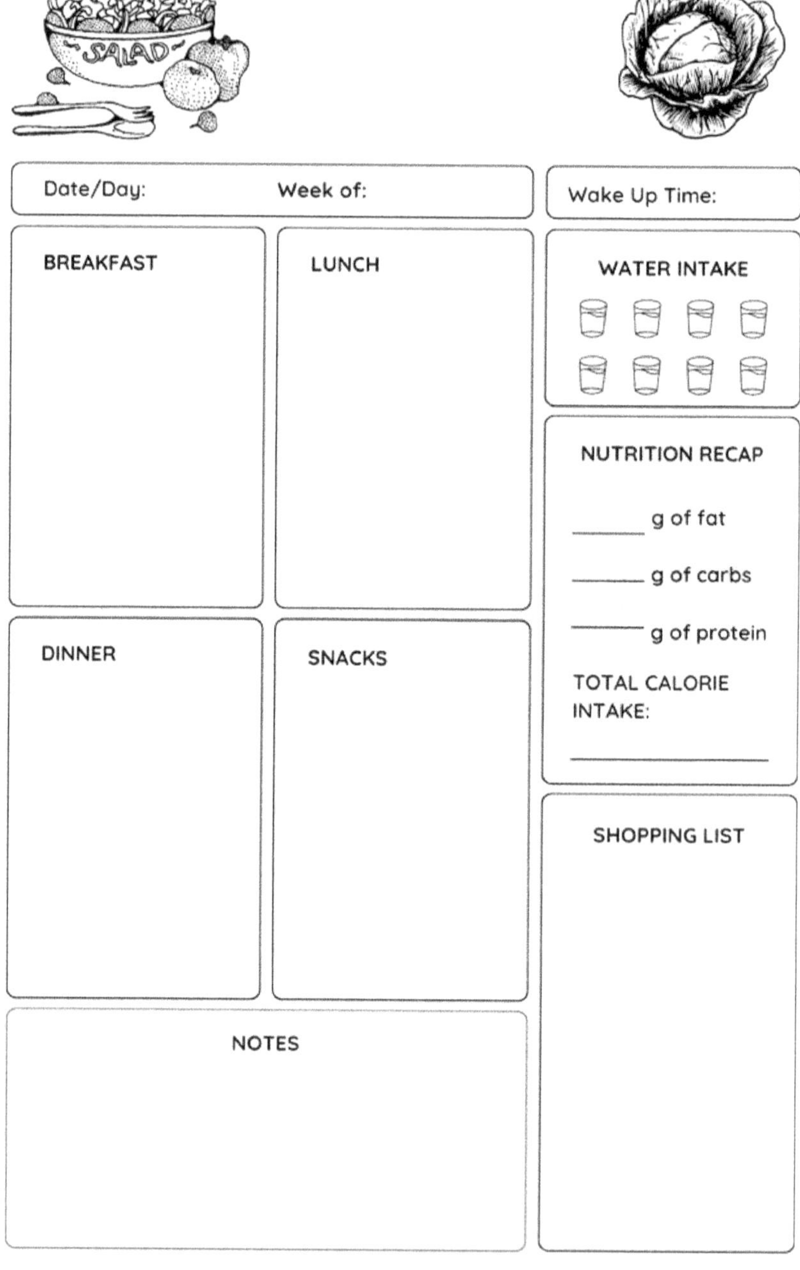


Date/Day:
Week of:
Wake Up Time:
BREAKFAST
LUNCH
WATER INTAKE
NUTRITION RECAP
_______ g of fat
_______ g of carbs
_______ g of protein
TOTAL CALORIE INTAKE:
DINNER
SNACKS
SHOPPING LIST
NOTES

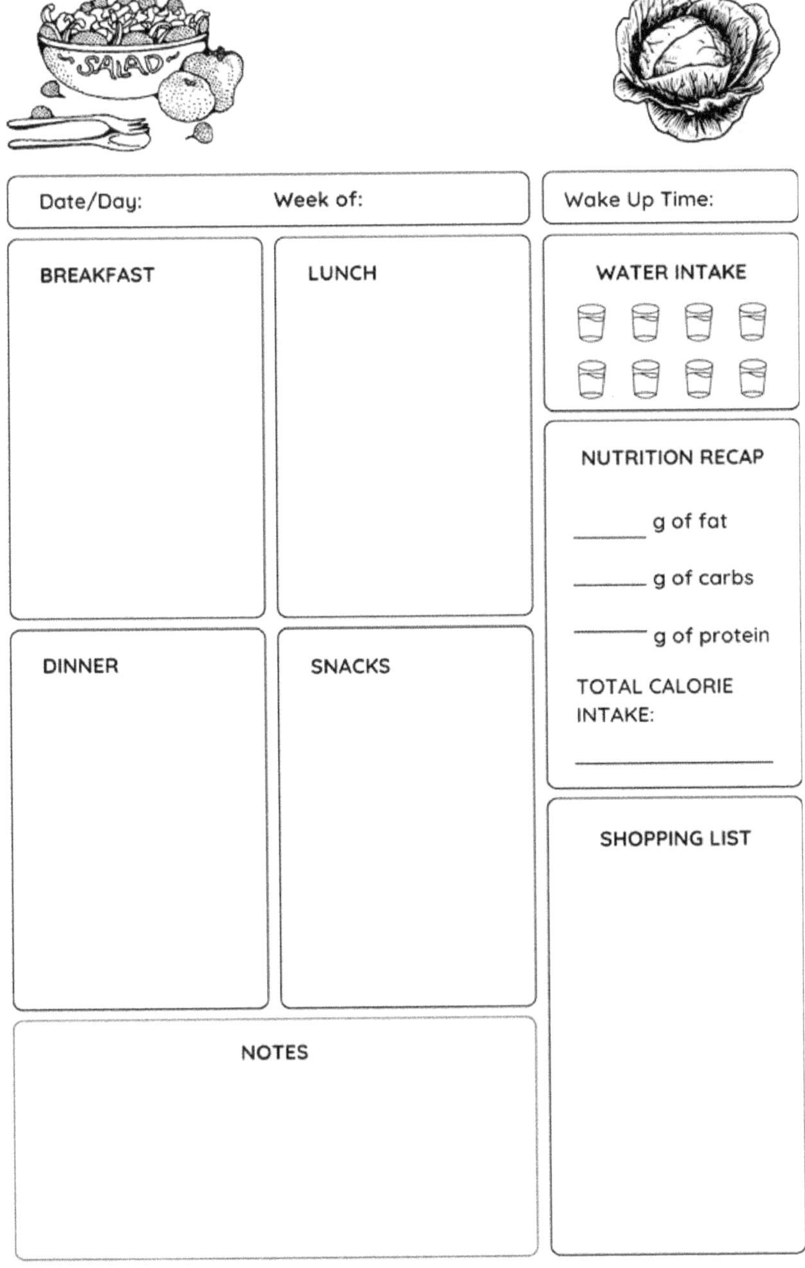

| Date/Day: | Week of: | Wake Up Time: |

**BREAKFAST**

**LUNCH**

**WATER INTAKE**

**NUTRITION RECAP**

______ g of fat

______ g of carbs

______ g of protein

**TOTAL CALORIE INTAKE:**

______

**DINNER**

**SNACKS**

**SHOPPING LIST**

**NOTES**

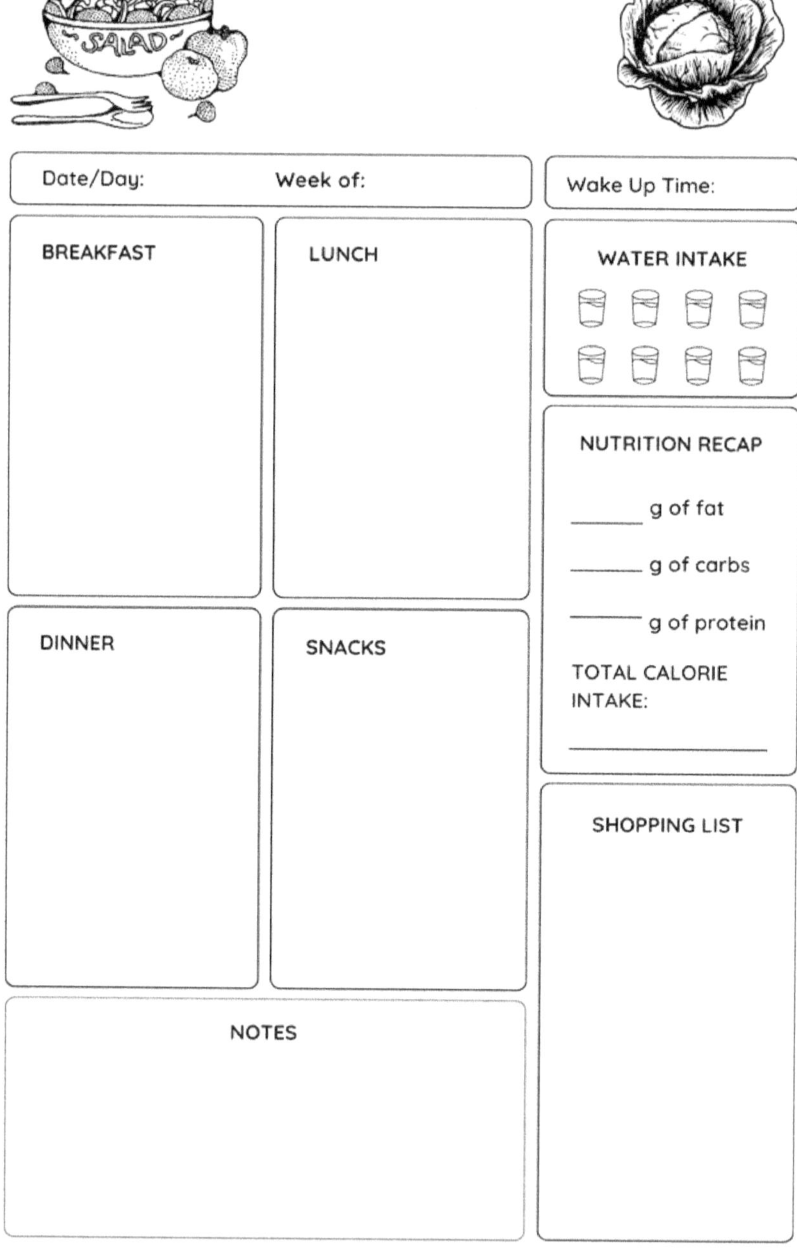


Date/Day:
Week of:
Wake Up Time:
BREAKFAST
LUNCH
WATER INTAKE
NUTRITION RECAP
_______ g of fat
_______ g of carbs
_______ g of protein
TOTAL CALORIE INTAKE:
DINNER
SNACKS
SHOPPING LIST
NOTES

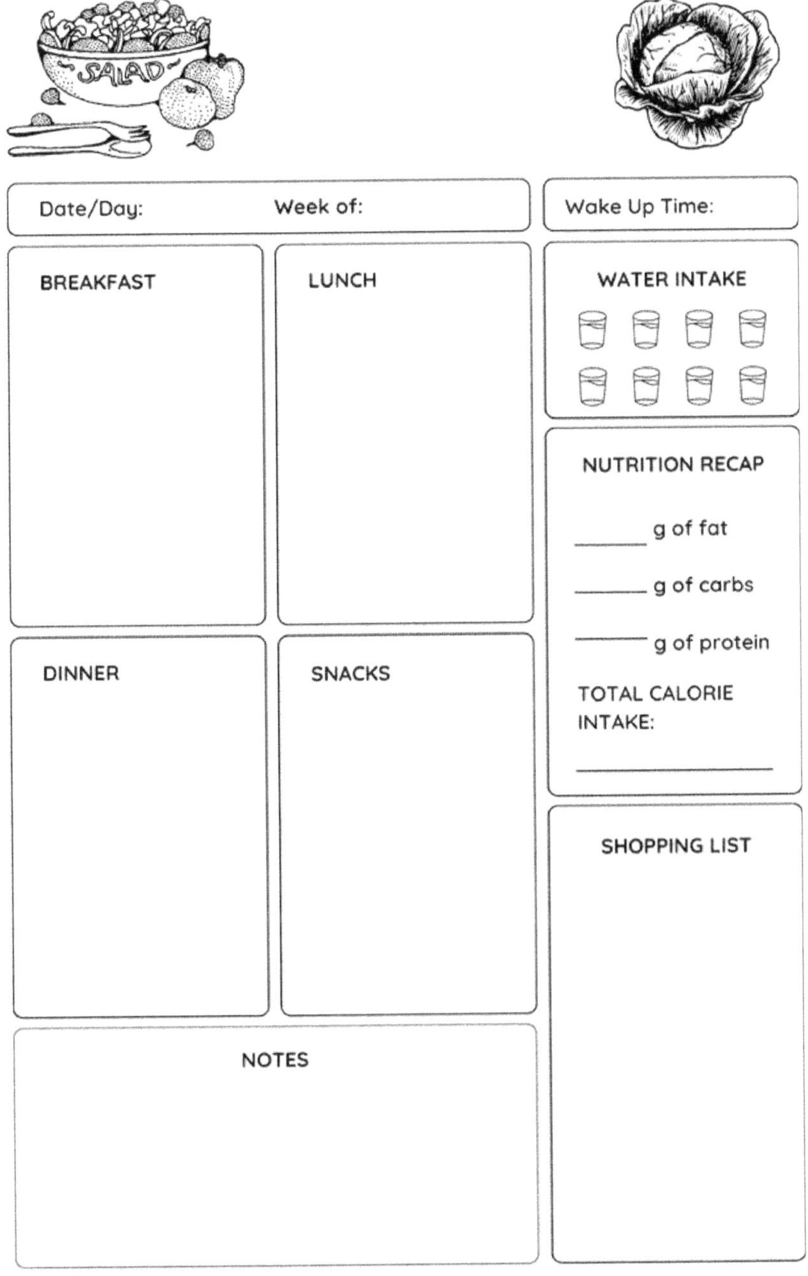


Date/Day:
Week of:
Wake Up Time:
BREAKFAST
LUNCH
WATER INTAKE
NUTRITION RECAP
_______ g of fat
_______ g of carbs
_______ g of protein
TOTAL CALORIE INTAKE:
DINNER
SNACKS
SHOPPING LIST
NOTES

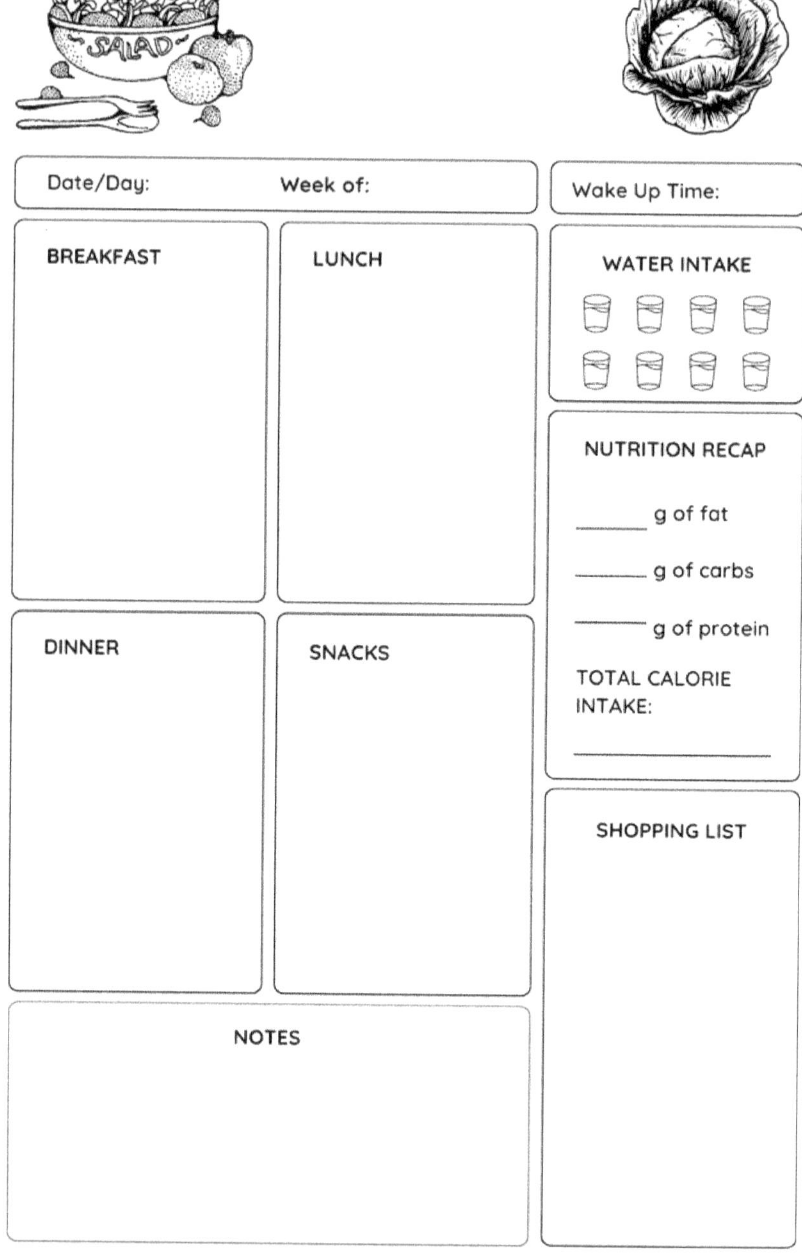

Date/Day:
Week of:
Wake Up Time:
BREAKFAST
LUNCH
WATER INTAKE
DINNER
SNACKS
NUTRITION RECAP
_______ g of fat
_______ g of carbs
_______ g of protein
TOTAL CALORIE INTAKE:
SHOPPING LIST
NOTES

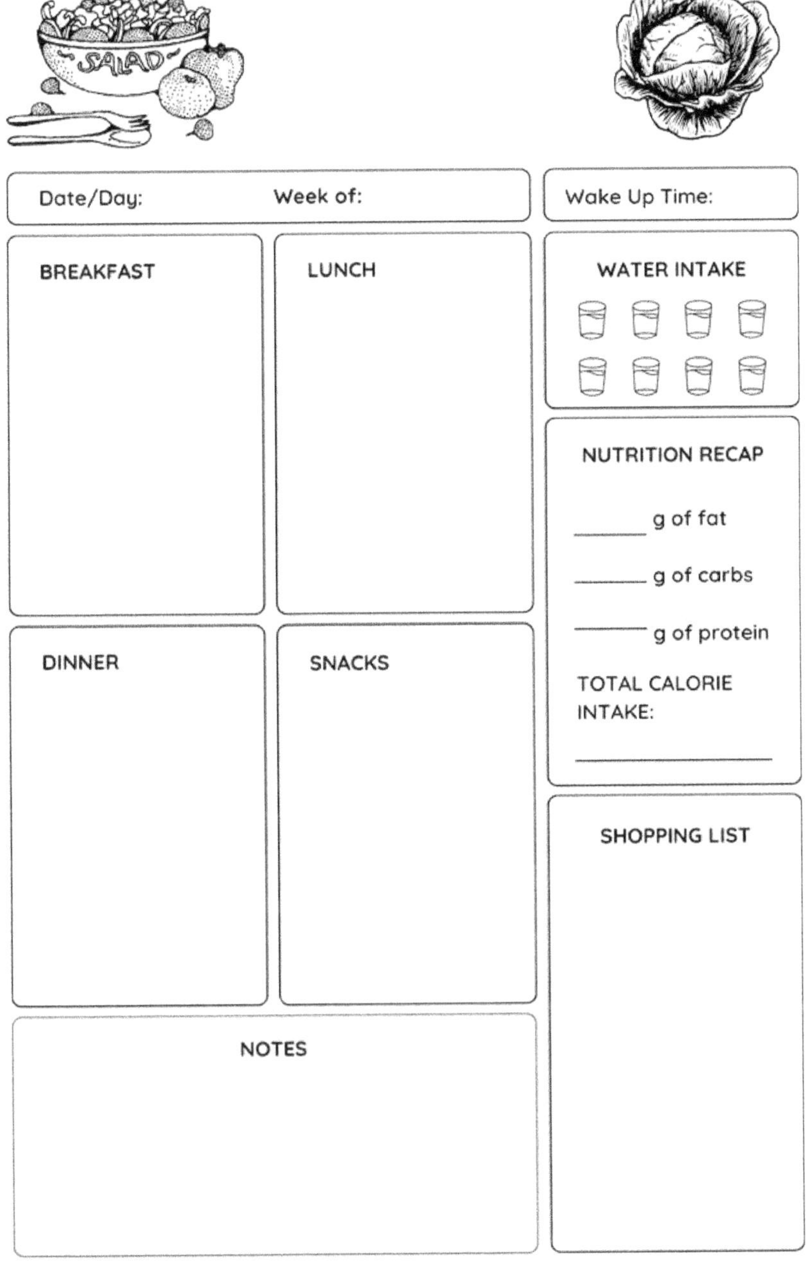

| Date/Day: | Week of: | Wake Up Time: |

**BREAKFAST**

**LUNCH**

**WATER INTAKE**

**NUTRITION RECAP**

_______ g of fat

_______ g of carbs

_______ g of protein

**TOTAL CALORIE INTAKE:**

_______________

**DINNER**

**SNACKS**

**SHOPPING LIST**

**NOTES**

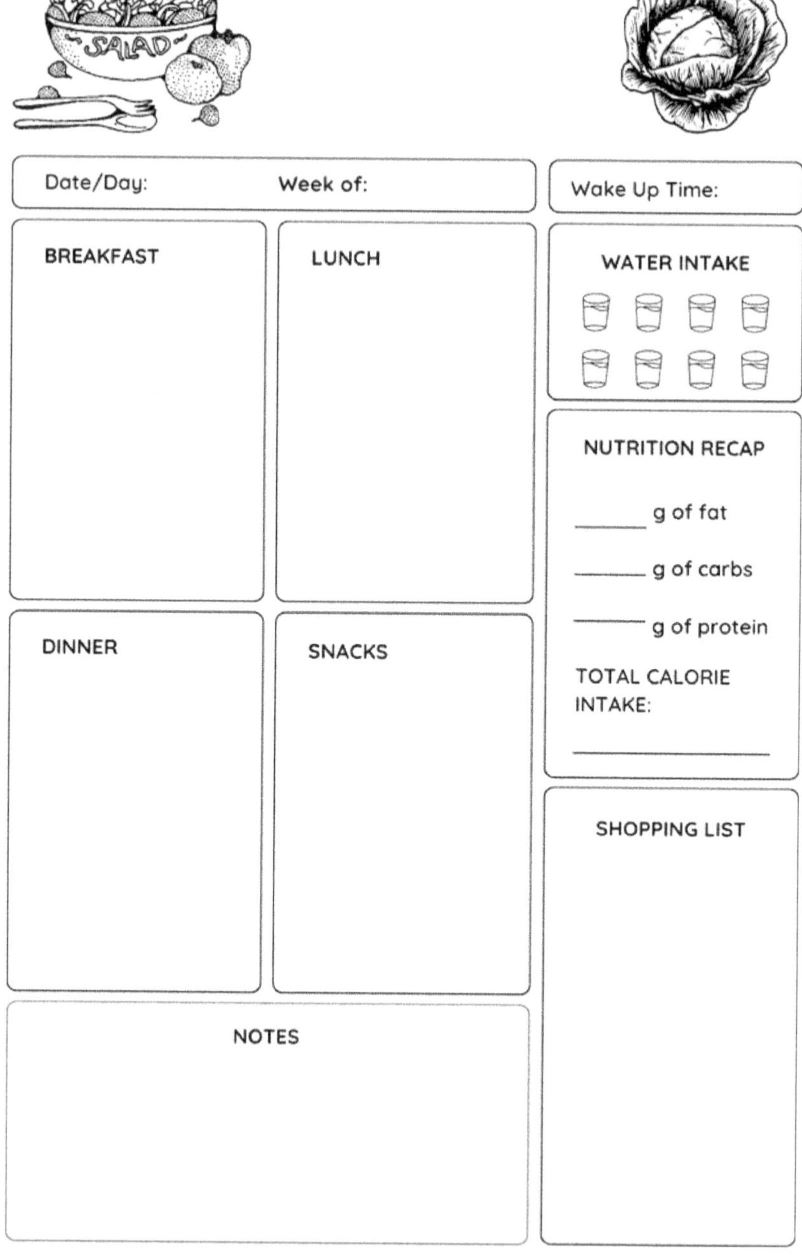

Date/Day:
Week of:
Wake Up Time:
BREAKFAST
LUNCH
WATER INTAKE
NUTRITION RECAP
_______ g of fat
_______ g of carbs
_______ g of protein
TOTAL CALORIE INTAKE:
DINNER
SNACKS
SHOPPING LIST
NOTES

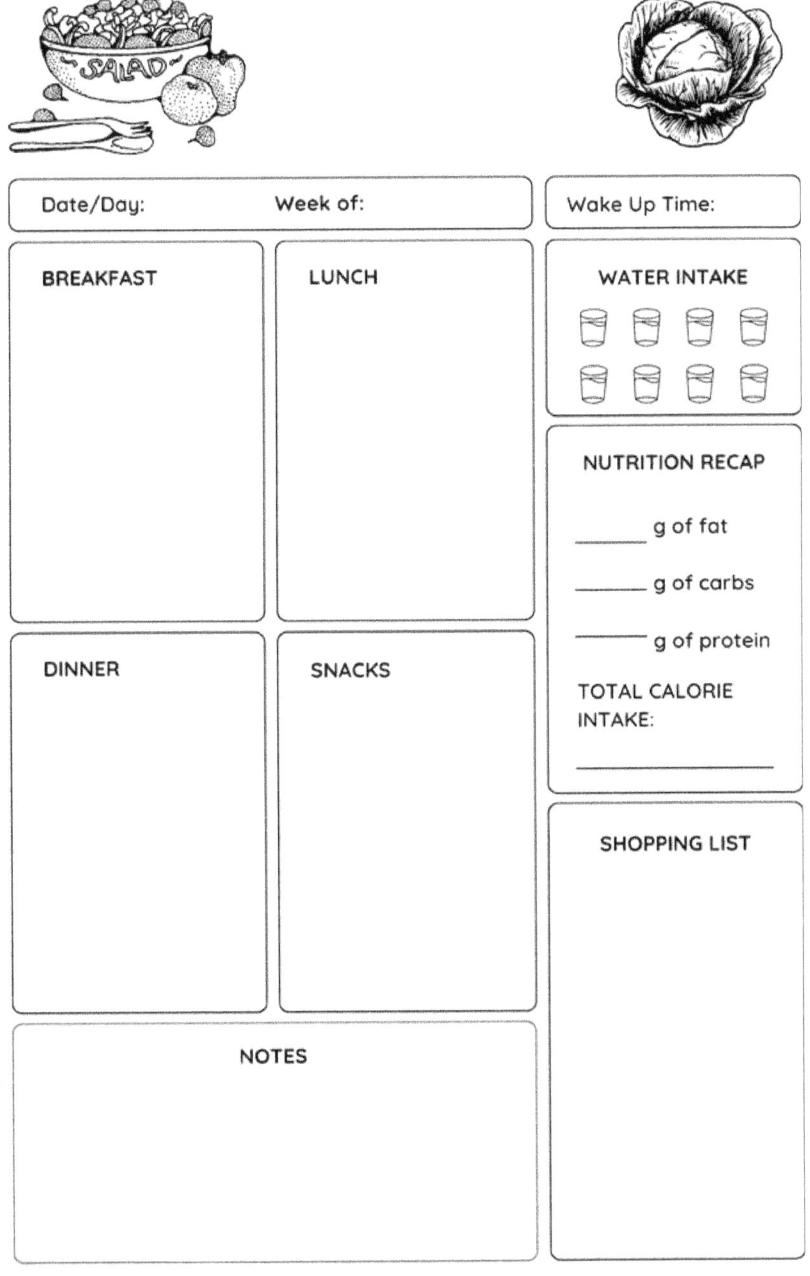


Date/Day:
Week of:
Wake Up Time:
BREAKFAST
LUNCH
WATER INTAKE
NUTRITION RECAP
_______ g of fat
_______ g of carbs
_______ g of protein
TOTAL CALORIE INTAKE:
DINNER
SNACKS
SHOPPING LIST
NOTES

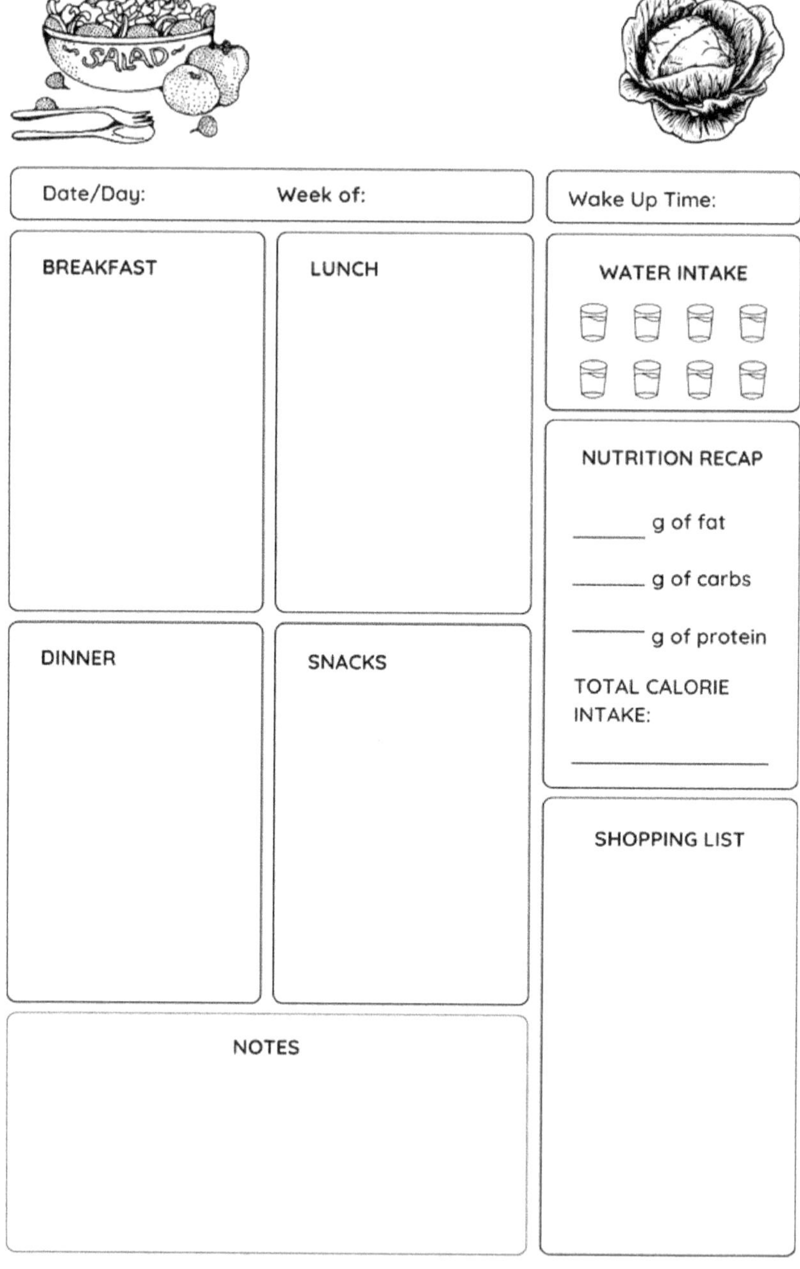

Date/Day:
Week of:
Wake Up Time:
BREAKFAST
LUNCH
WATER INTAKE
NUTRITION RECAP
_______ g of fat
_______ g of carbs
_______ g of protein
TOTAL CALORIE INTAKE:
DINNER
SNACKS
SHOPPING LIST
NOTES

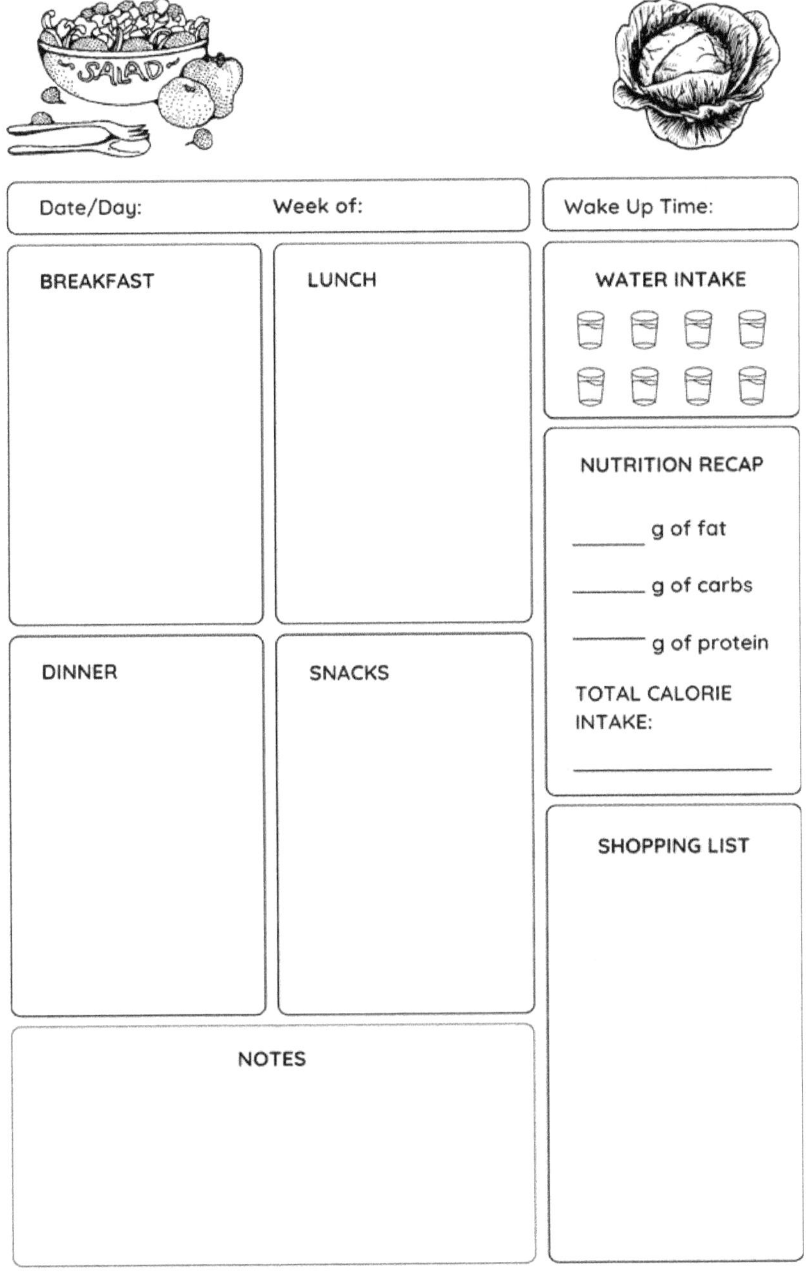

| Date/Day: | Week of: | Wake Up Time: |

**BREAKFAST**

**LUNCH**

**WATER INTAKE**

**NUTRITION RECAP**

_______ g of fat

_______ g of carbs

_______ g of protein

**TOTAL CALORIE INTAKE:**

_______________

**DINNER**

**SNACKS**

**SHOPPING LIST**

**NOTES**

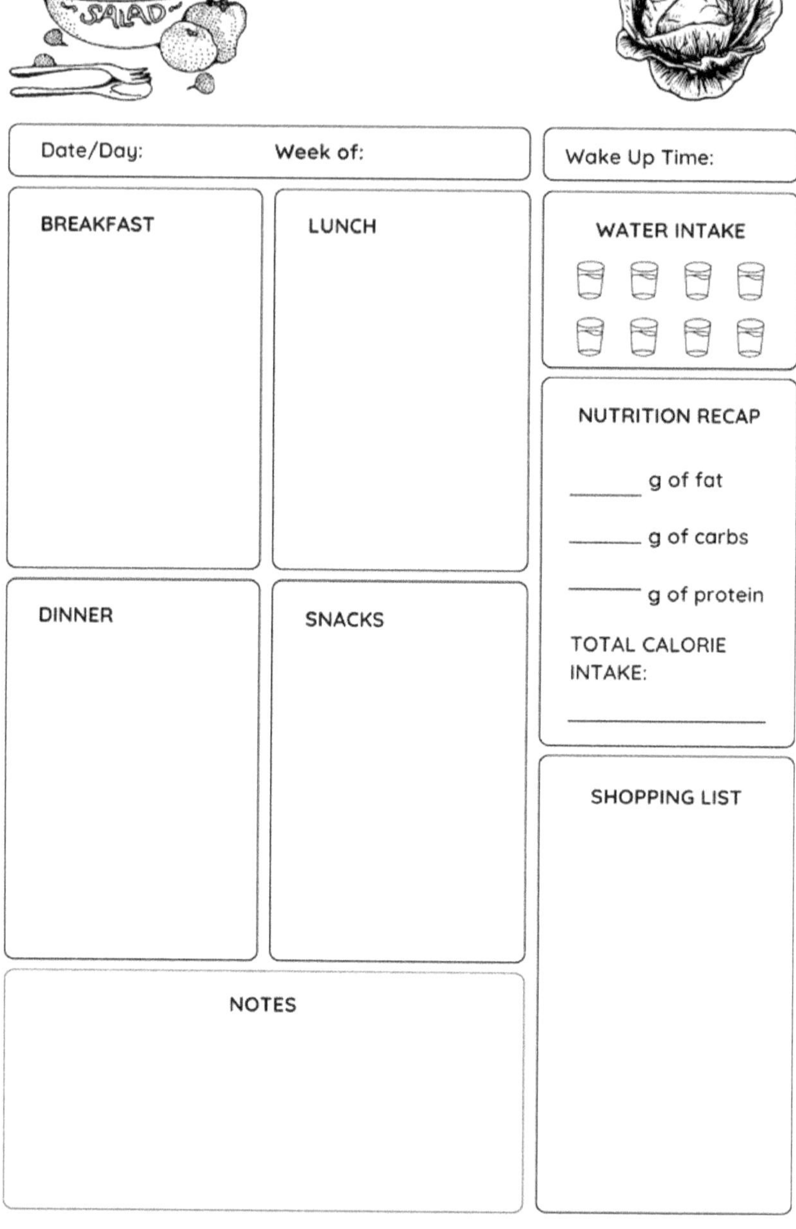

SALAD

Date/Day:
Week of:
Wake Up Time:

BREAKFAST

LUNCH

WATER INTAKE

NUTRITION RECAP

_______ g of fat

_______ g of carbs

_______ g of protein

DINNER

SNACKS

TOTAL CALORIE
INTAKE:

NOTES

SHOPPING LIST

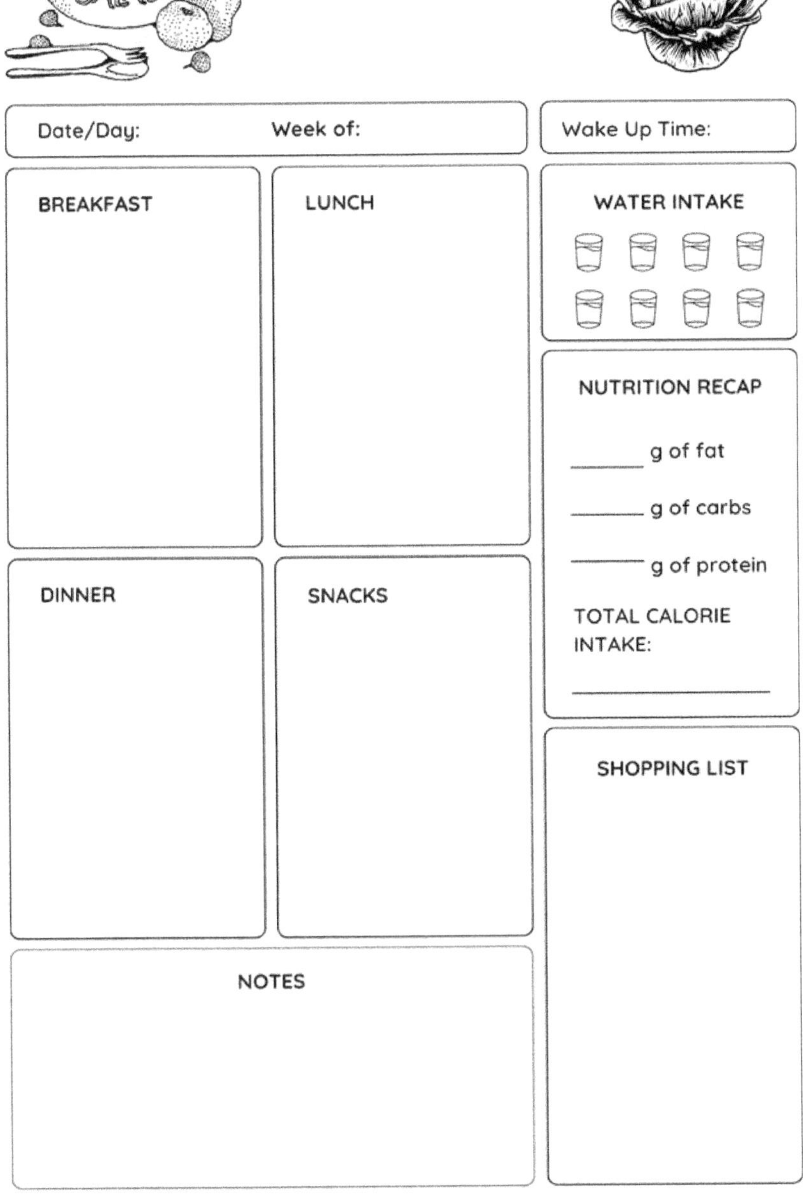



Date/Day:  Week of:

Wake Up Time:

BREAKFAST

LUNCH

WATER INTAKE

NUTRITION RECAP

_________ g of fat

_________ g of carbs

_________ g of protein

TOTAL CALORIE INTAKE:

_____________________

DINNER

SNACKS

SHOPPING LIST

NOTES

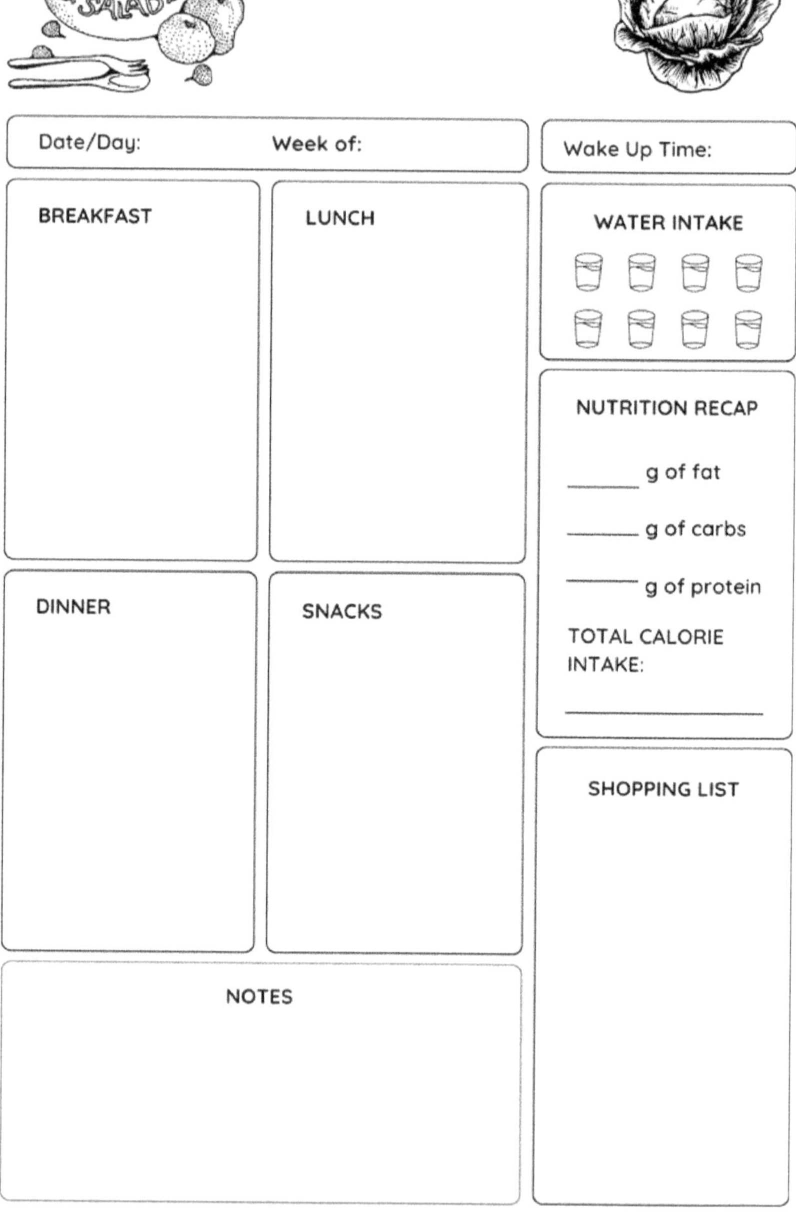


Date/Day:
Week of:
Wake Up Time:
BREAKFAST
LUNCH
WATER INTAKE
NUTRITION RECAP
_______ g of fat
_______ g of carbs
_______ g of protein
TOTAL CALORIE INTAKE:
DINNER
SNACKS
SHOPPING LIST
NOTES

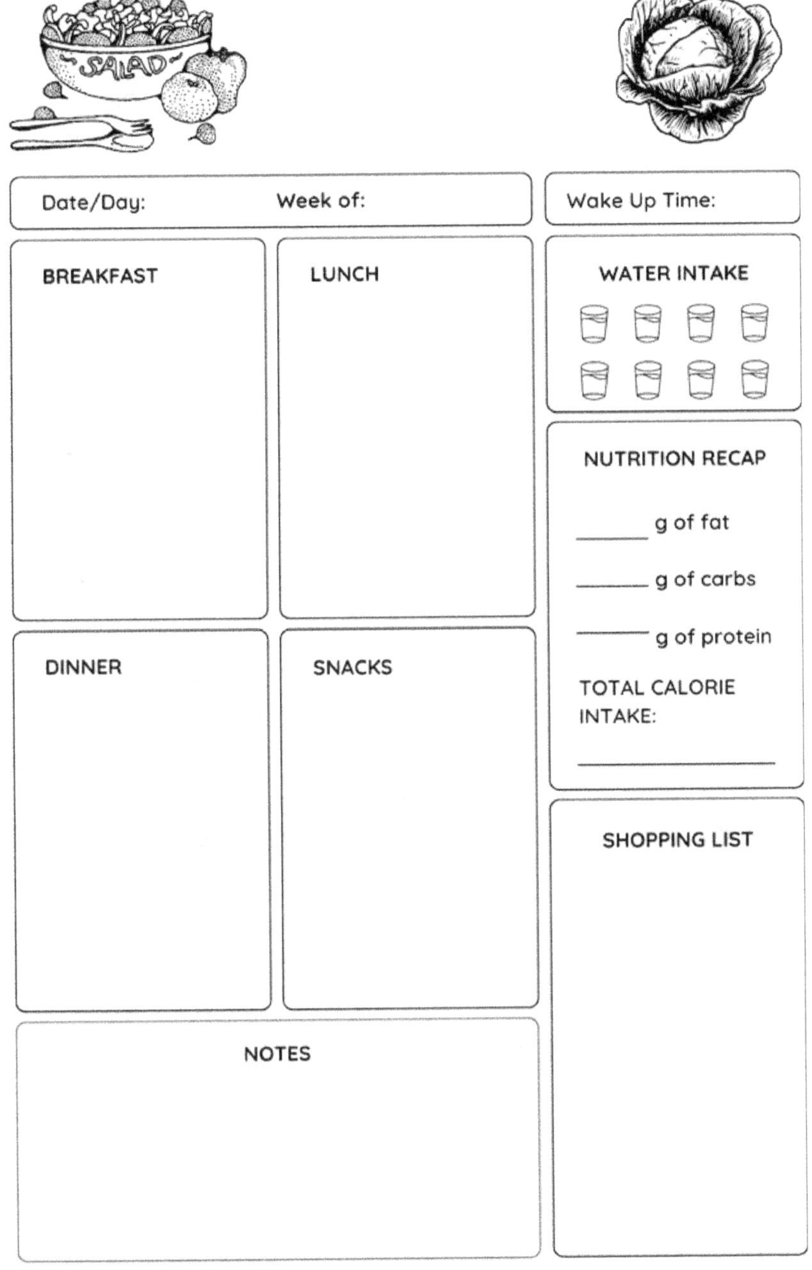



| Date/Day: | Week of: | Wake Up Time: |

**BREAKFAST**

**LUNCH**

**WATER INTAKE**

**NUTRITION RECAP**

_______ g of fat

_______ g of carbs

_______ g of protein

**TOTAL CALORIE INTAKE:**

**DINNER**

**SNACKS**

**SHOPPING LIST**

**NOTES**

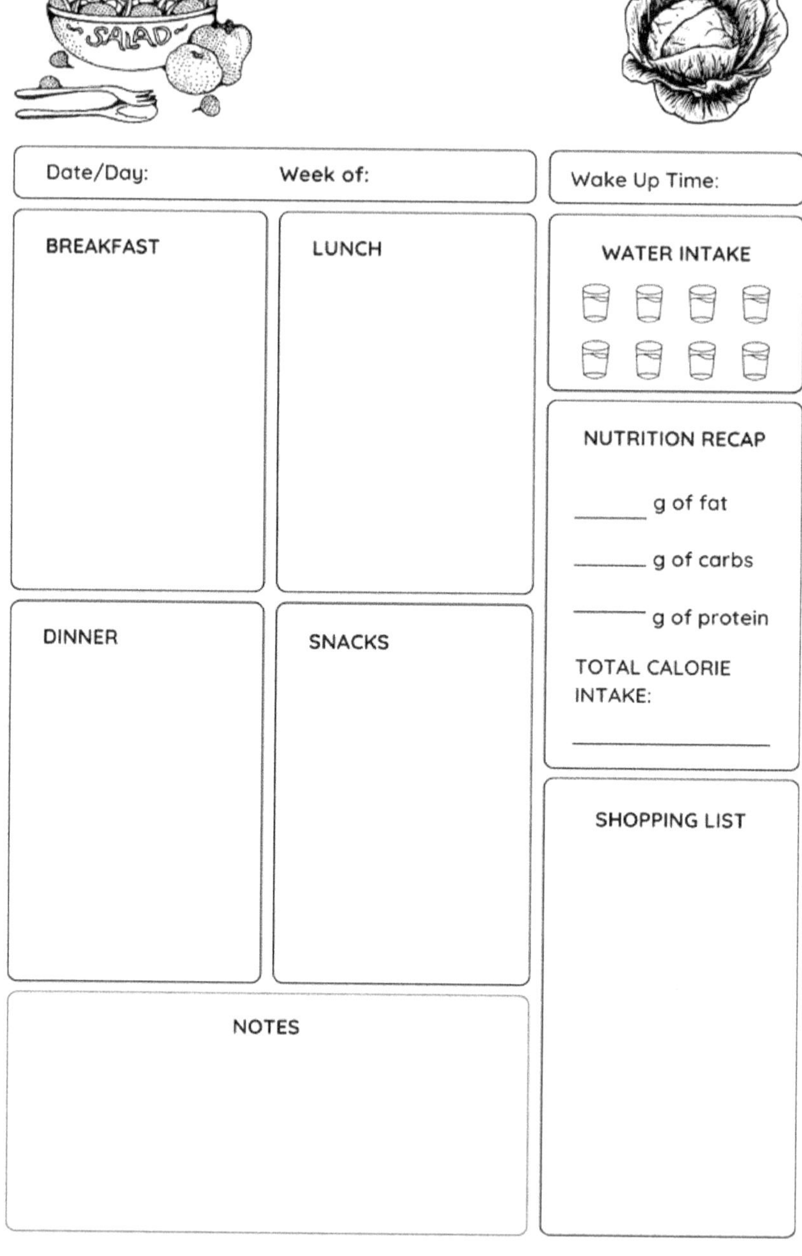

| Date/Day: | Week of: | Wake Up Time: |

**BREAKFAST**

**LUNCH**

**WATER INTAKE**

**NUTRITION RECAP**

_______ g of fat

_______ g of carbs

_______ g of protein

**TOTAL CALORIE INTAKE:**

**DINNER**

**SNACKS**

**SHOPPING LIST**

**NOTES**

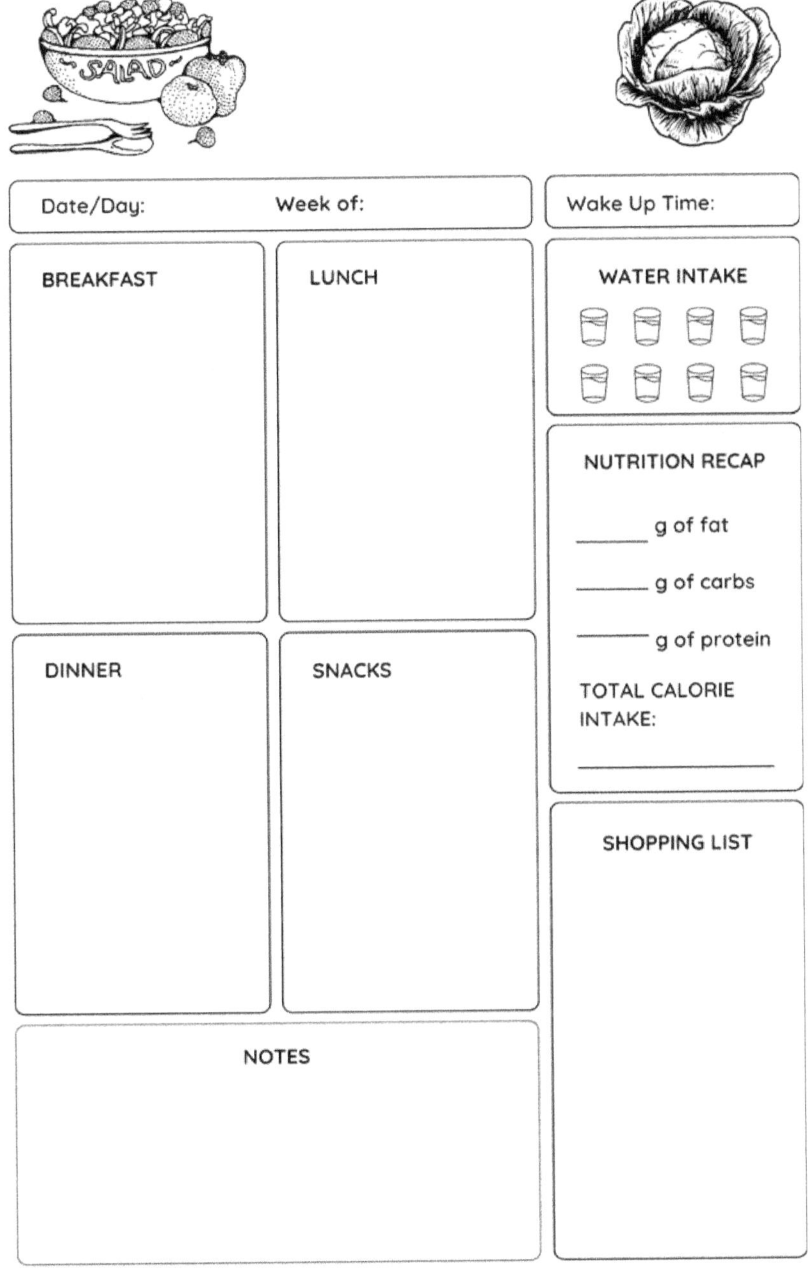


Date/Day:
Week of:
Wake Up Time:
BREAKFAST
LUNCH
WATER INTAKE
NUTRITION RECAP
_______ g of fat
_______ g of carbs
_______ g of protein
TOTAL CALORIE INTAKE:
DINNER
SNACKS
SHOPPING LIST
NOTES

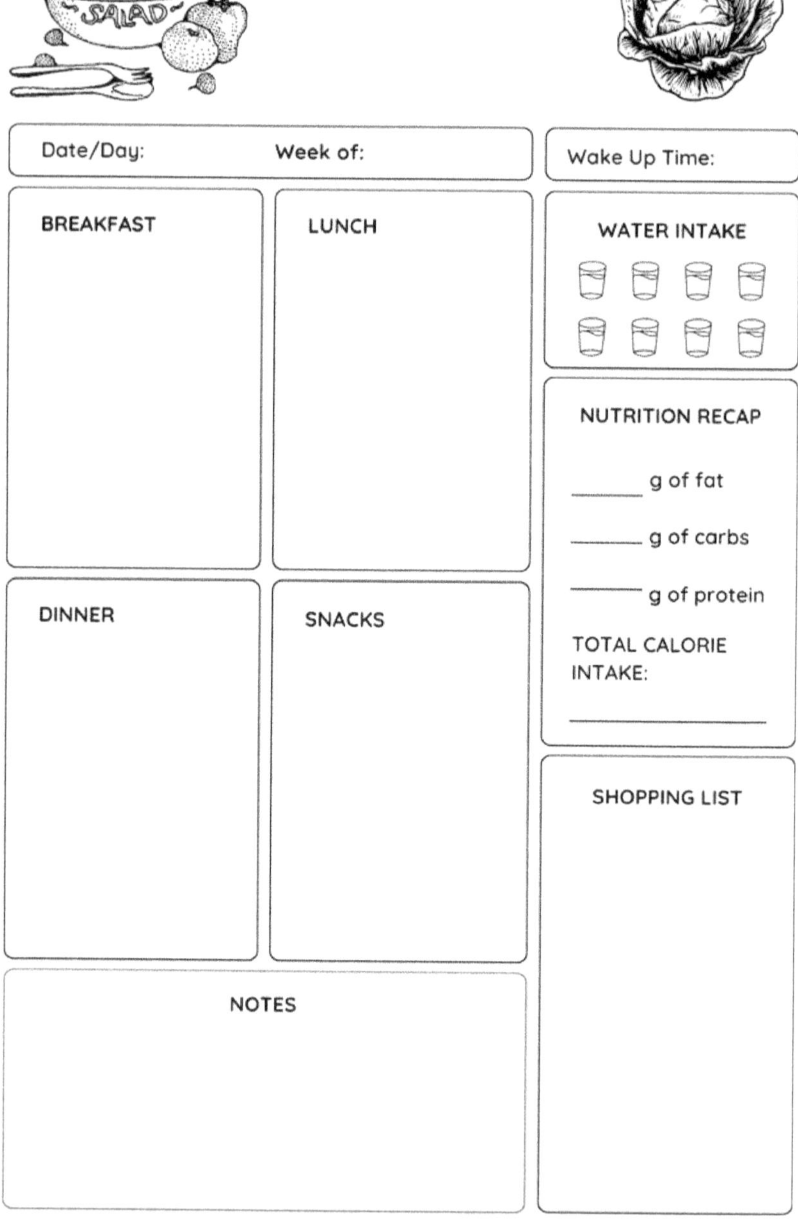


Date/Day:
Week of:
Wake Up Time:
BREAKFAST
LUNCH
WATER INTAKE
NUTRITION RECAP
_______ g of fat
_______ g of carbs
_______ g of protein
TOTAL CALORIE INTAKE:
DINNER
SNACKS
SHOPPING LIST
NOTES

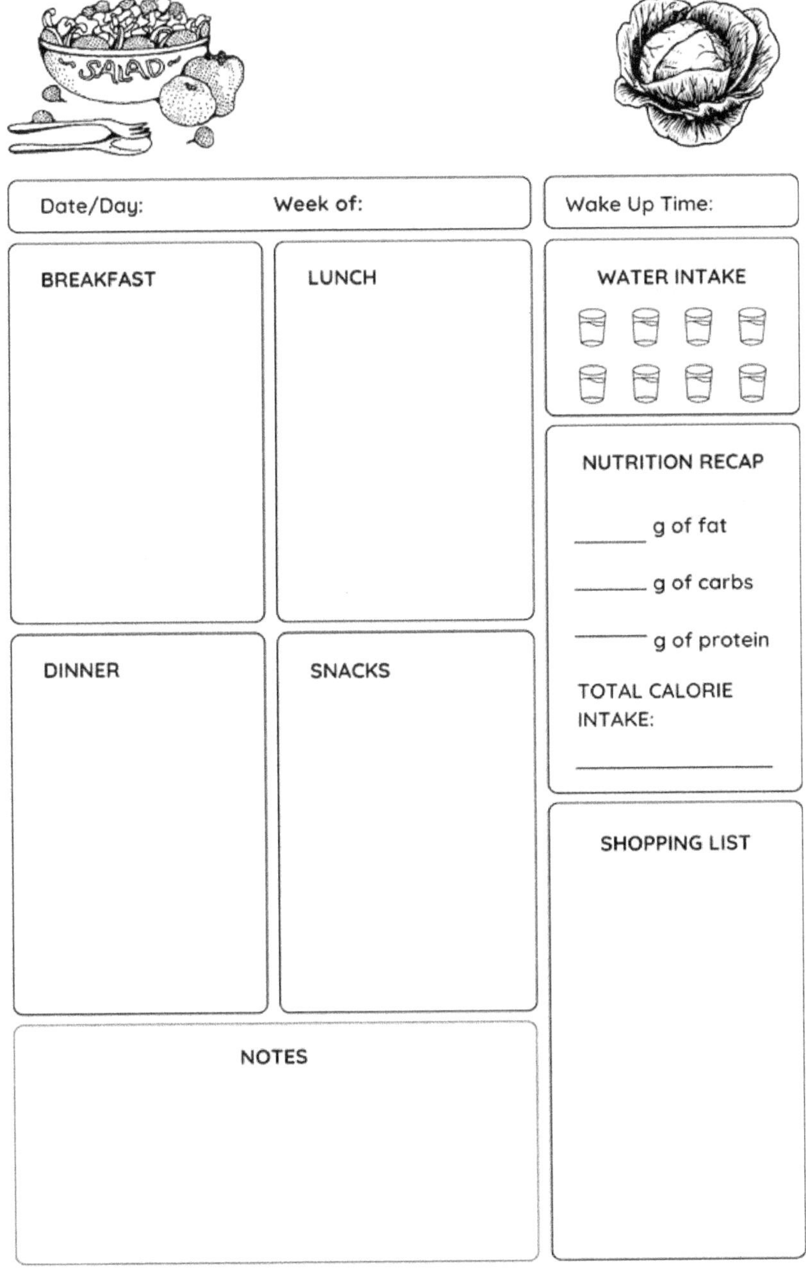

Date/Day:
Week of:
Wake Up Time:
BREAKFAST
LUNCH
WATER INTAKE
NUTRITION RECAP
_______ g of fat
_______ g of carbs
_______ g of protein
TOTAL CALORIE INTAKE:
DINNER
SNACKS
SHOPPING LIST
NOTES

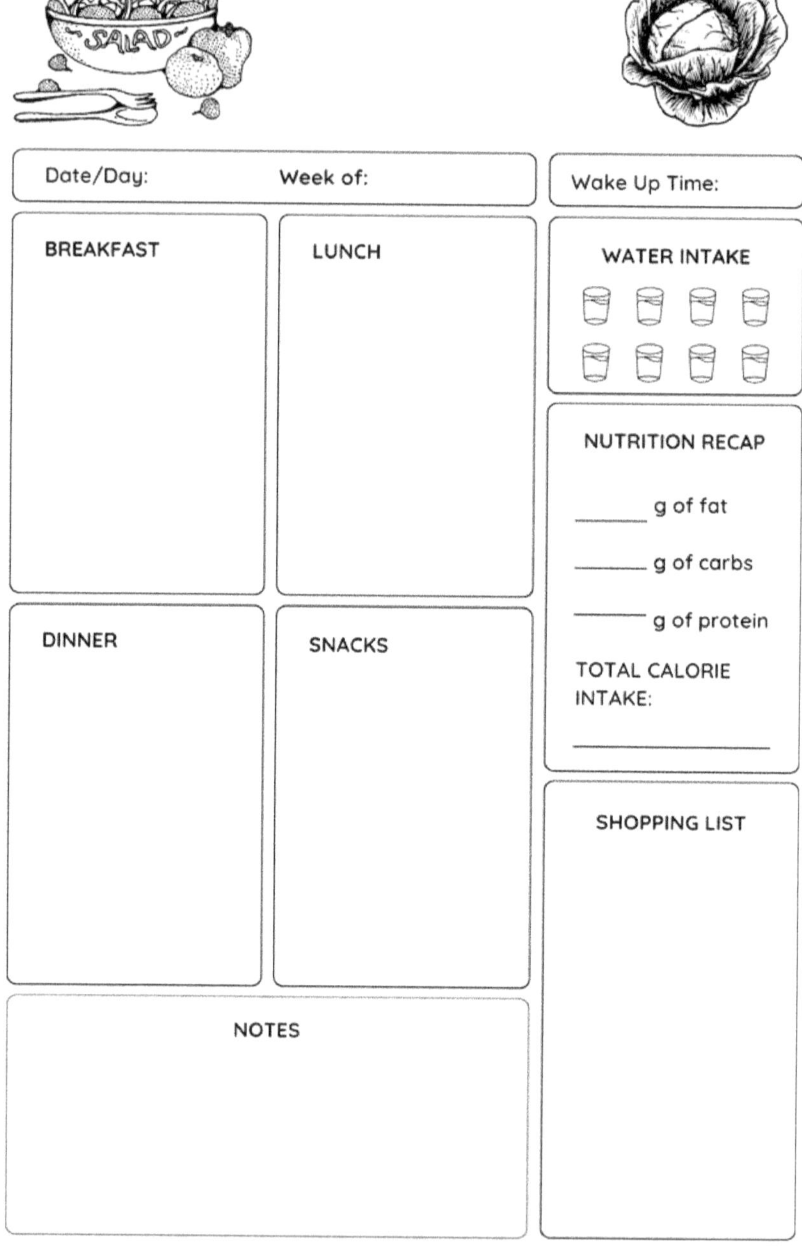


Date/Day:
Week of:
Wake Up Time:
BREAKFAST
LUNCH
WATER INTAKE
NUTRITION RECAP
_______ g of fat
_______ g of carbs
_______ g of protein
TOTAL CALORIE INTAKE:
DINNER
SNACKS
SHOPPING LIST
NOTES

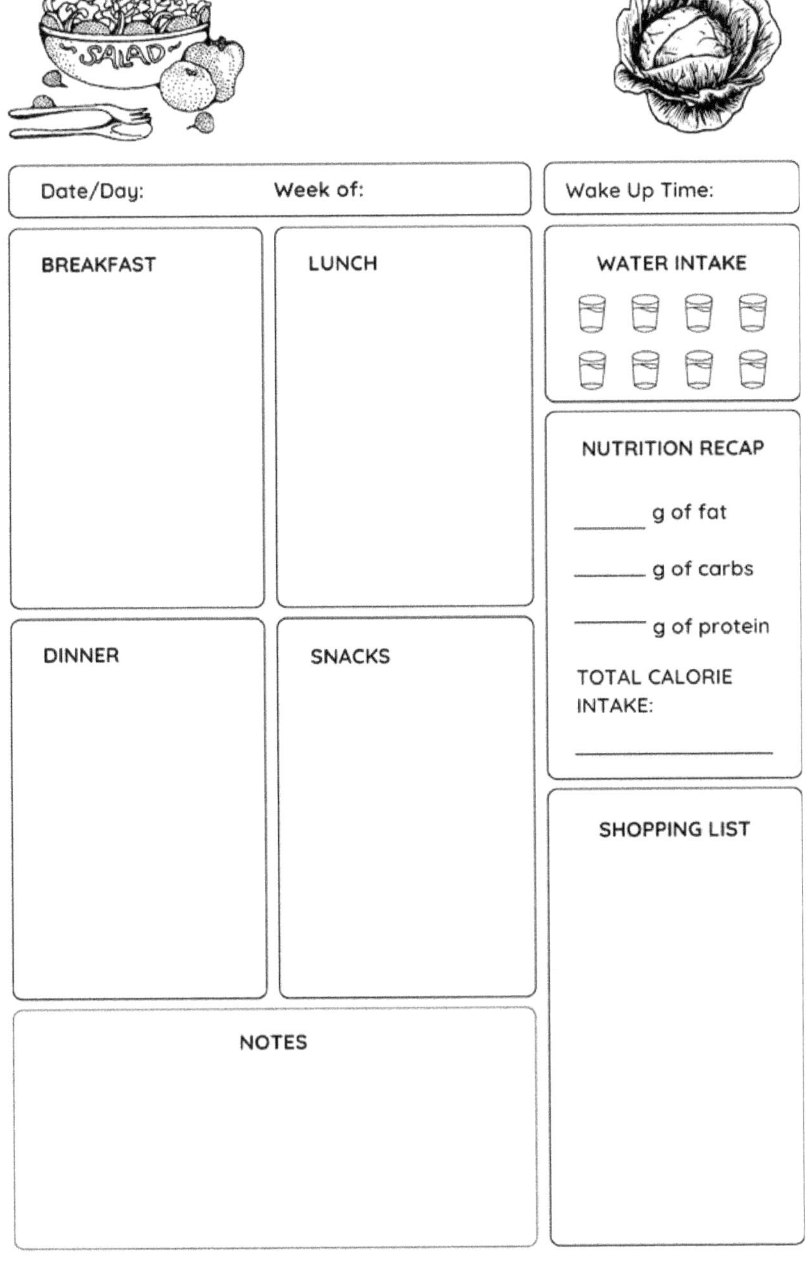


Date/Day:     Week of:

Wake Up Time:

BREAKFAST

LUNCH

WATER INTAKE

NUTRITION RECAP

_______ g of fat

_______ g of carbs

_______ g of protein

TOTAL CALORIE INTAKE:

DINNER

SNACKS

SHOPPING LIST

NOTES

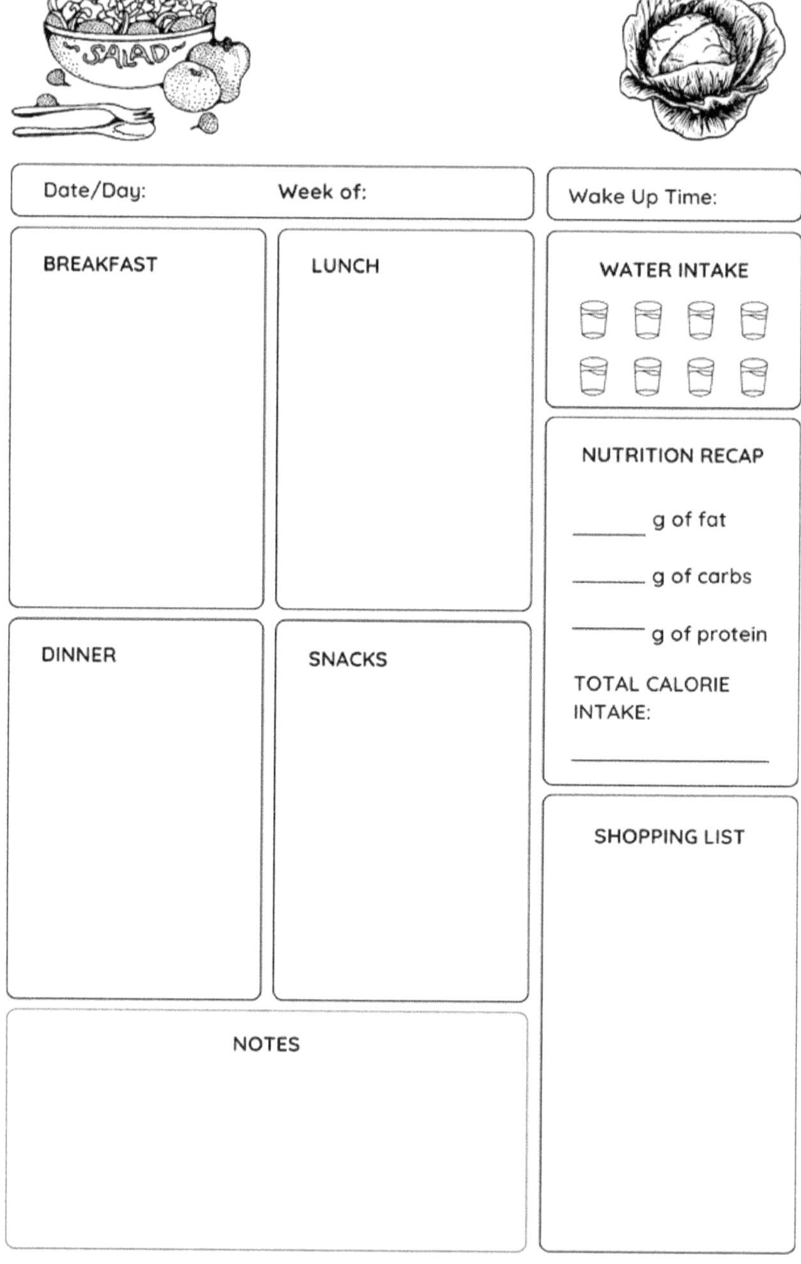

Date/Day:
Week of:
Wake Up Time:
BREAKFAST
LUNCH
WATER INTAKE
NUTRITION RECAP
_______ g of fat
_______ g of carbs
_______ g of protein
TOTAL CALORIE INTAKE:
DINNER
SNACKS
SHOPPING LIST
NOTES

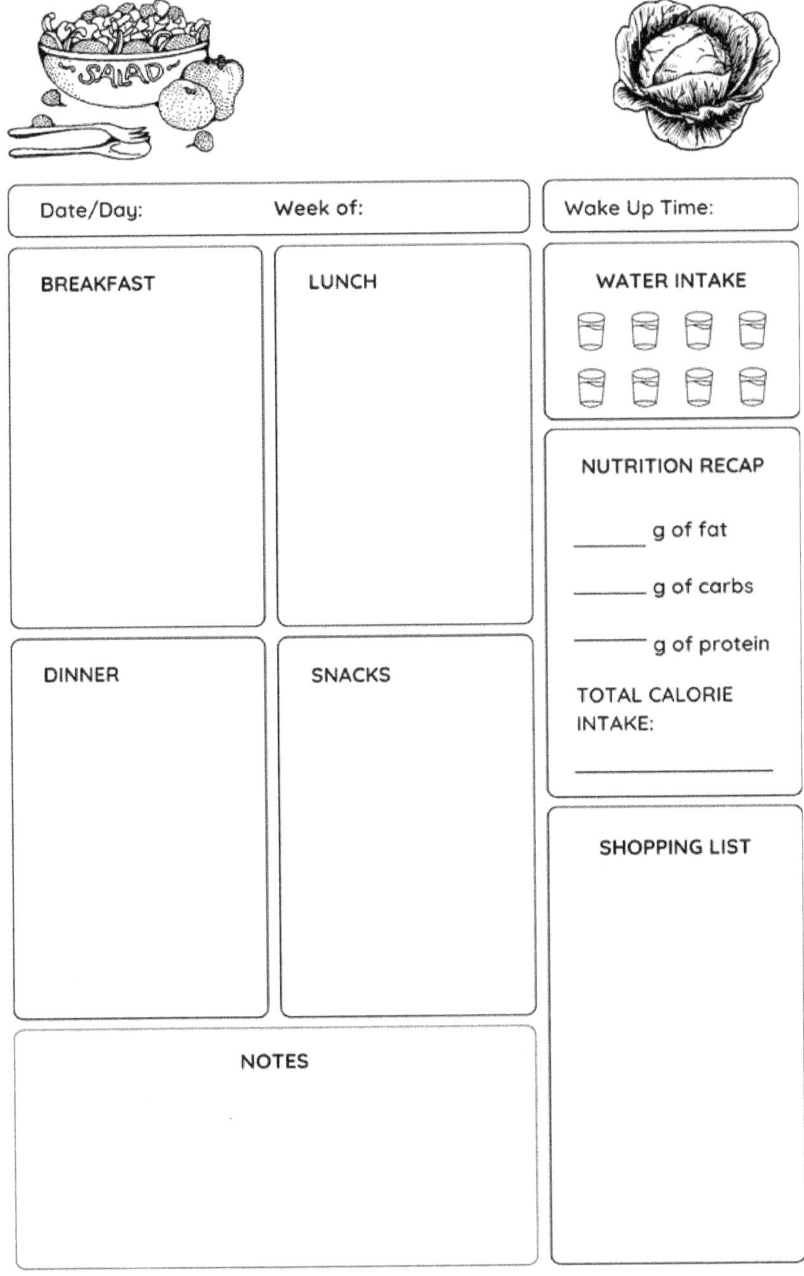


Date/Day:                Week of:
Wake Up Time:
BREAKFAST
LUNCH
WATER INTAKE
NUTRITION RECAP
_______ g of fat
_______ g of carbs
_______ g of protein
TOTAL CALORIE INTAKE:
_______________
DINNER
SNACKS
SHOPPING LIST
NOTES

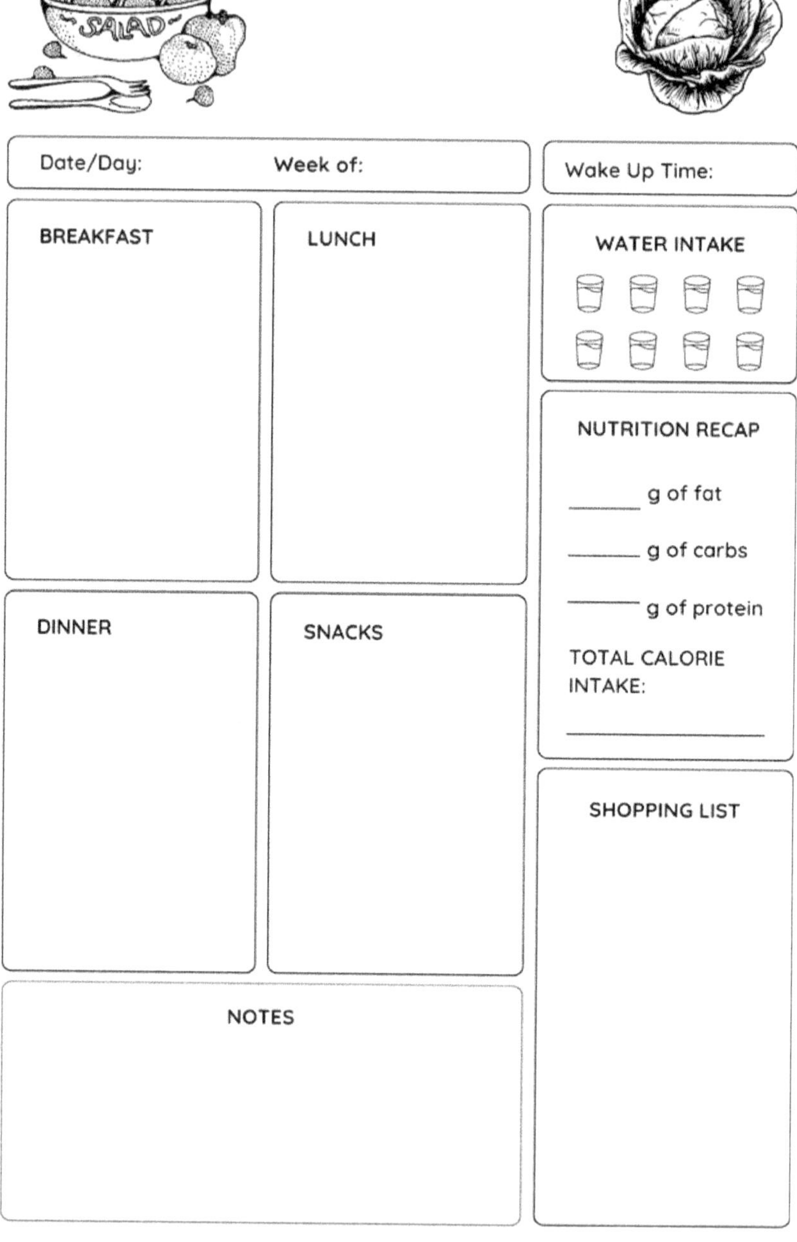

Date/Day:
Week of:
Wake Up Time:
BREAKFAST
LUNCH
WATER INTAKE
NUTRITION RECAP
_______ g of fat
_______ g of carbs
_______ g of protein
TOTAL CALORIE INTAKE:
DINNER
SNACKS
SHOPPING LIST
NOTES

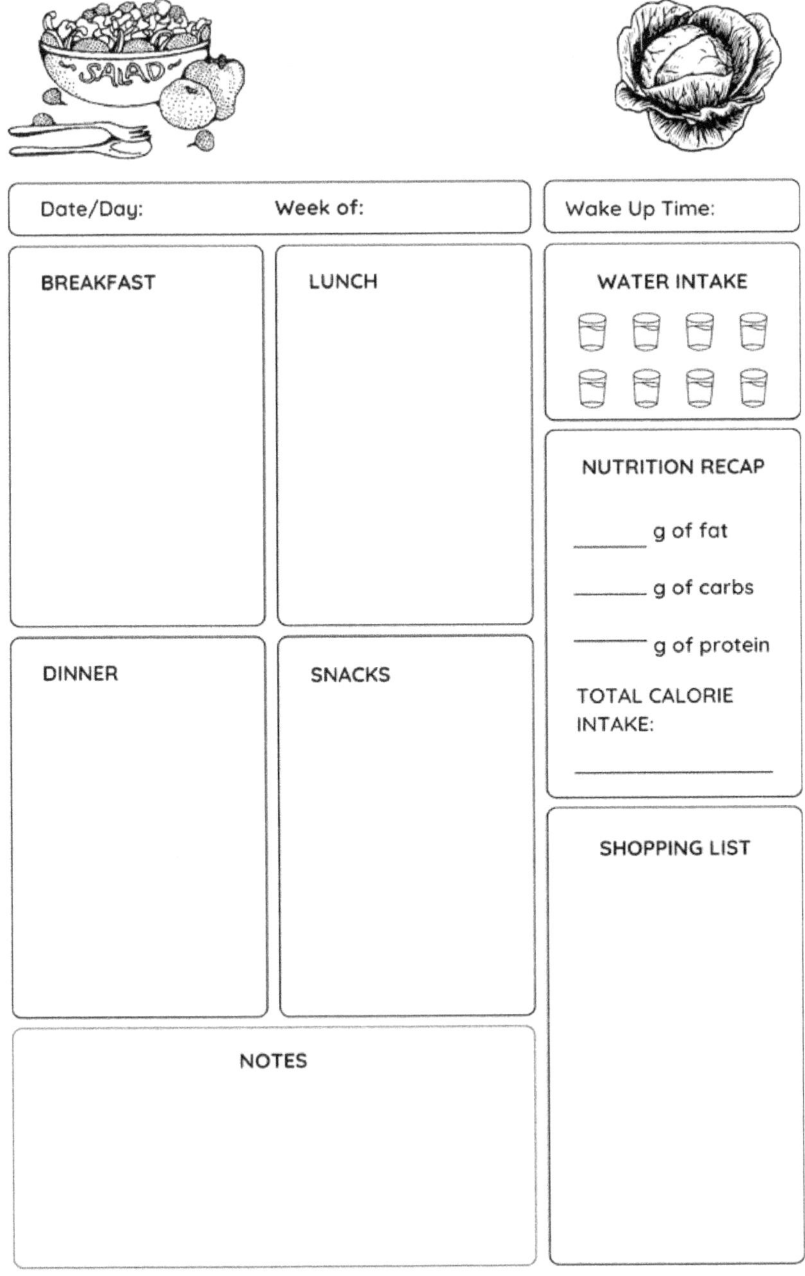

| Date/Day: | Week of: | Wake Up Time: |

**BREAKFAST**

**LUNCH**

**WATER INTAKE**

**NUTRITION RECAP**

_______ g of fat

_______ g of carbs

_______ g of protein

**TOTAL CALORIE INTAKE:**

_______________

**DINNER**

**SNACKS**

**SHOPPING LIST**

**NOTES**

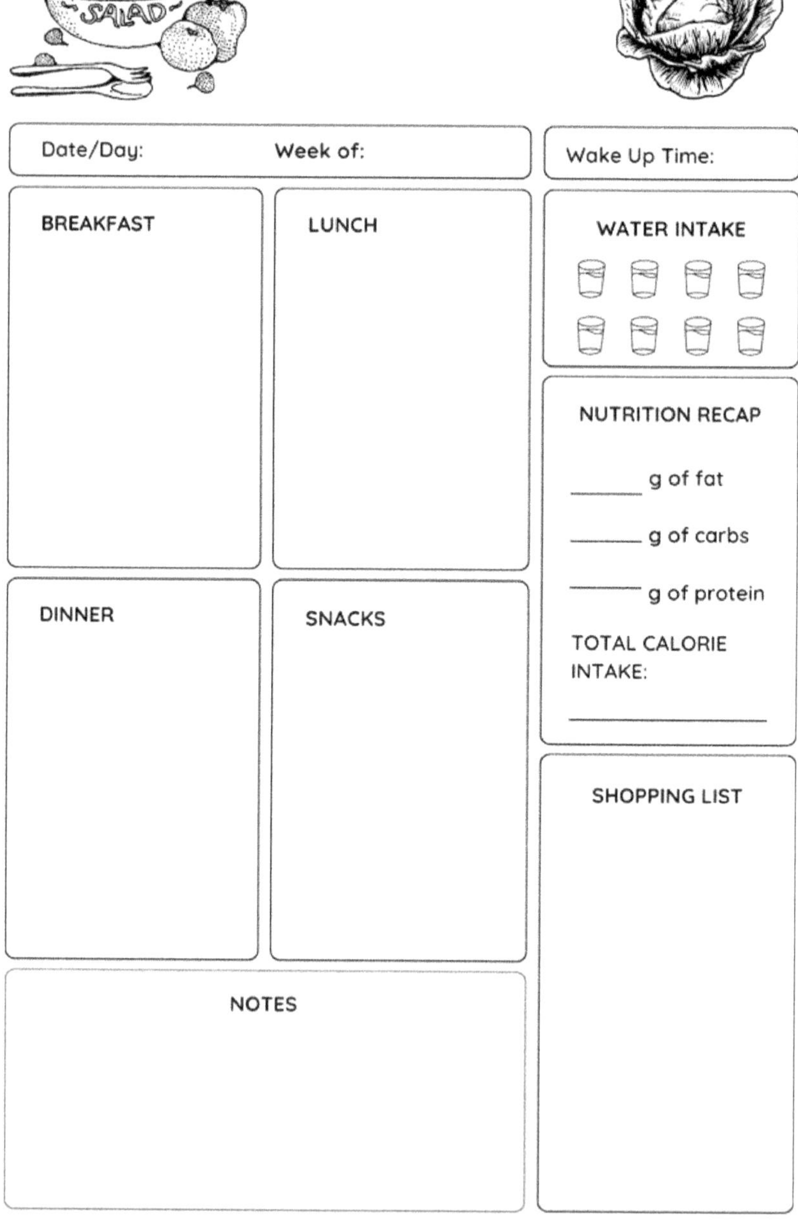


Date/Day:
Week of:
Wake Up Time:
BREAKFAST
LUNCH
WATER INTAKE
NUTRITION RECAP
_______ g of fat
_______ g of carbs
_______ g of protein
TOTAL CALORIE INTAKE:
DINNER
SNACKS
SHOPPING LIST
NOTES

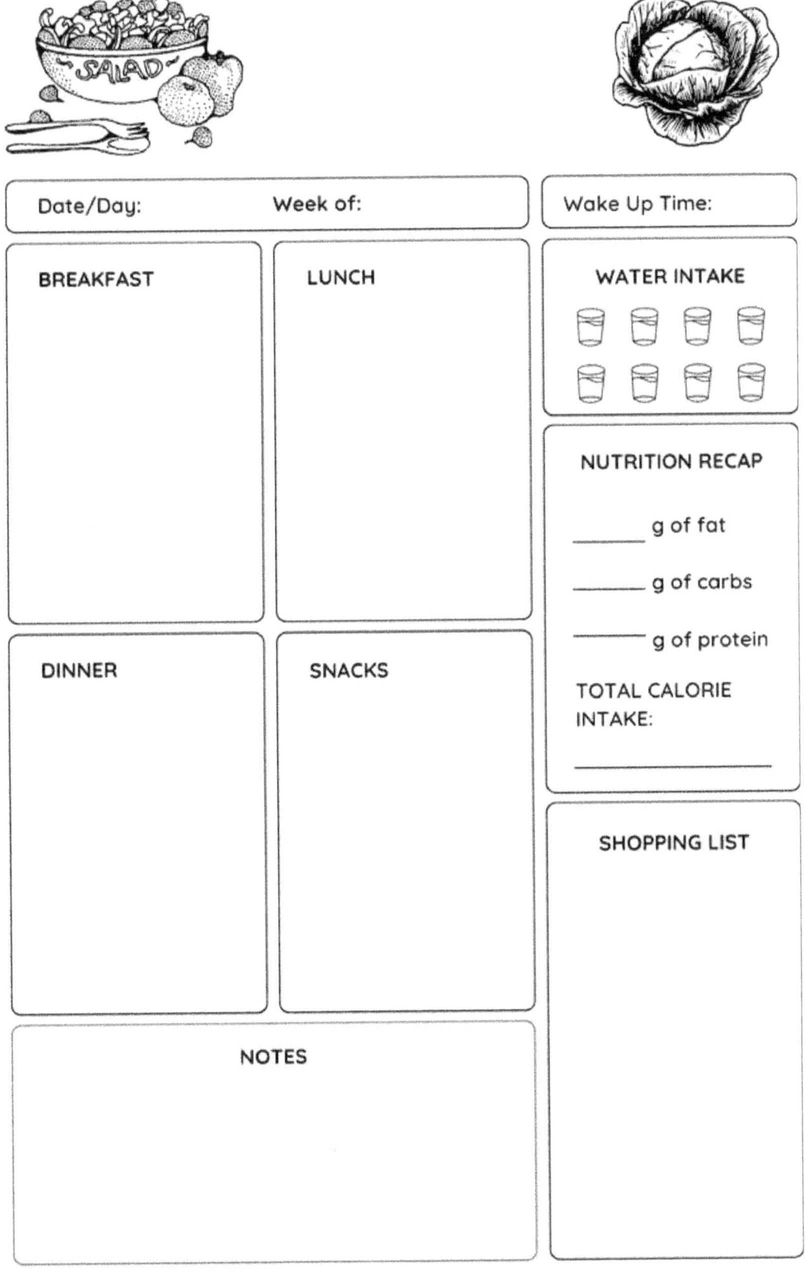

Date/Day:          Week of:

Wake Up Time:

BREAKFAST

LUNCH

WATER INTAKE

NUTRITION RECAP

________ g of fat

________ g of carbs

________ g of protein

TOTAL CALORIE INTAKE:

________

DINNER

SNACKS

SHOPPING LIST

NOTES

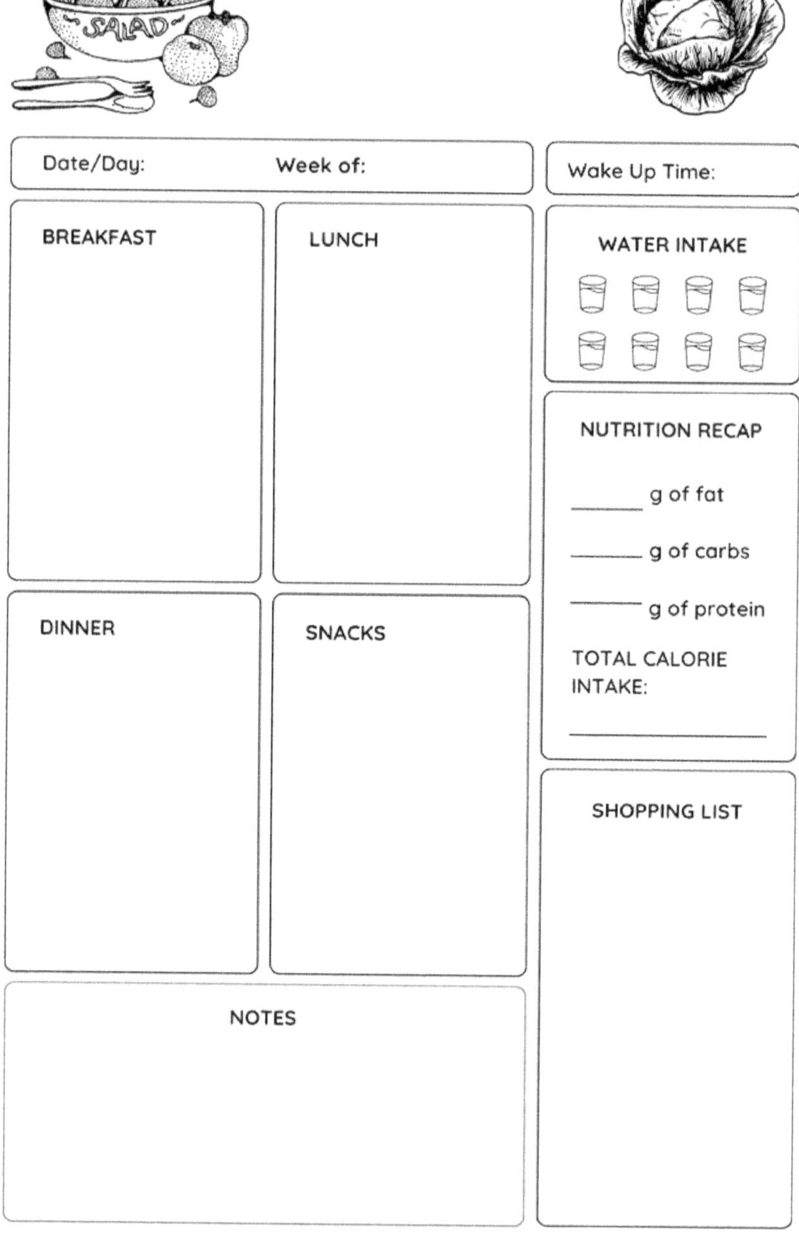
Date/Day:
Week of:
Wake Up Time:
BREAKFAST
LUNCH
WATER INTAKE
NUTRITION RECAP
_______ g of fat
_______ g of carbs
_______ g of protein
TOTAL CALORIE INTAKE:
DINNER
SNACKS
SHOPPING LIST
NOTES

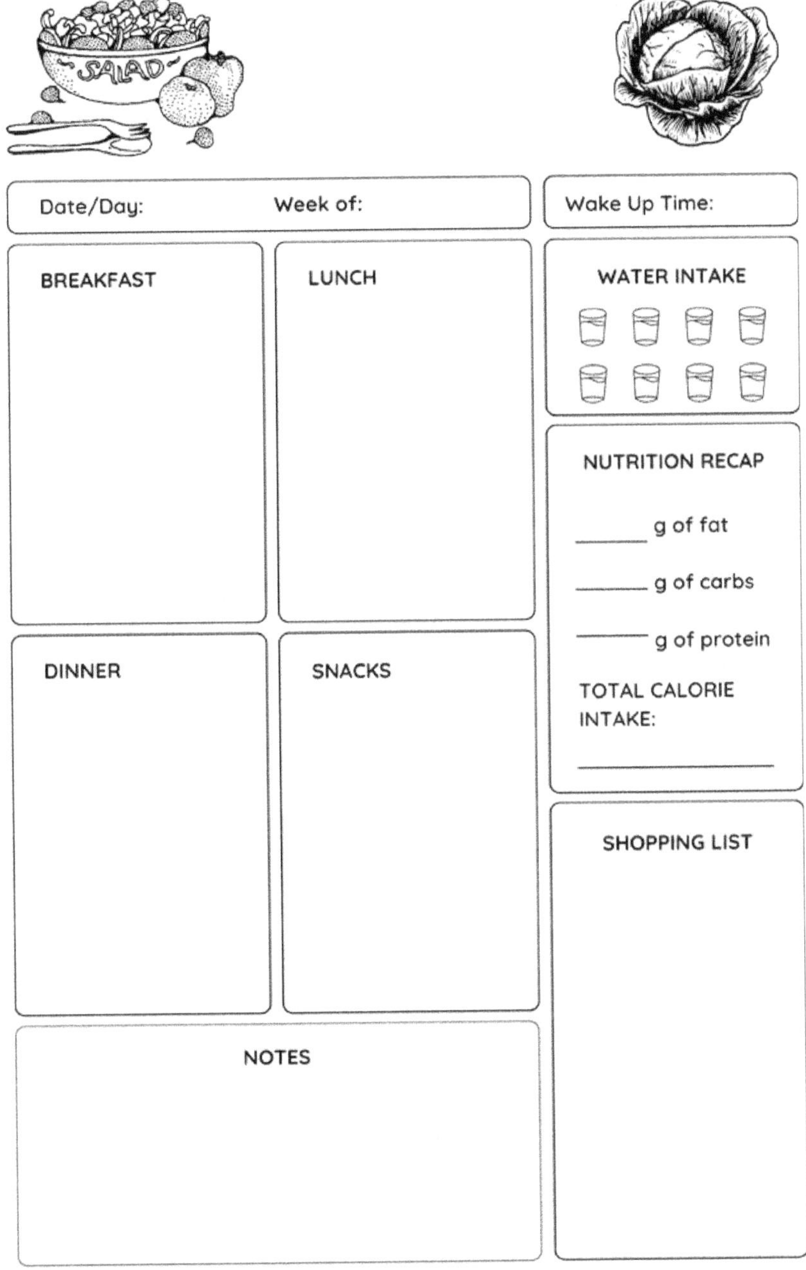

| Date/Day: | Week of: | Wake Up Time: |

**BREAKFAST**

**LUNCH**

**WATER INTAKE**

**NUTRITION RECAP**

________ g of fat

________ g of carbs

________ g of protein

**TOTAL CALORIE INTAKE:**

**DINNER**

**SNACKS**

**SHOPPING LIST**

**NOTES**

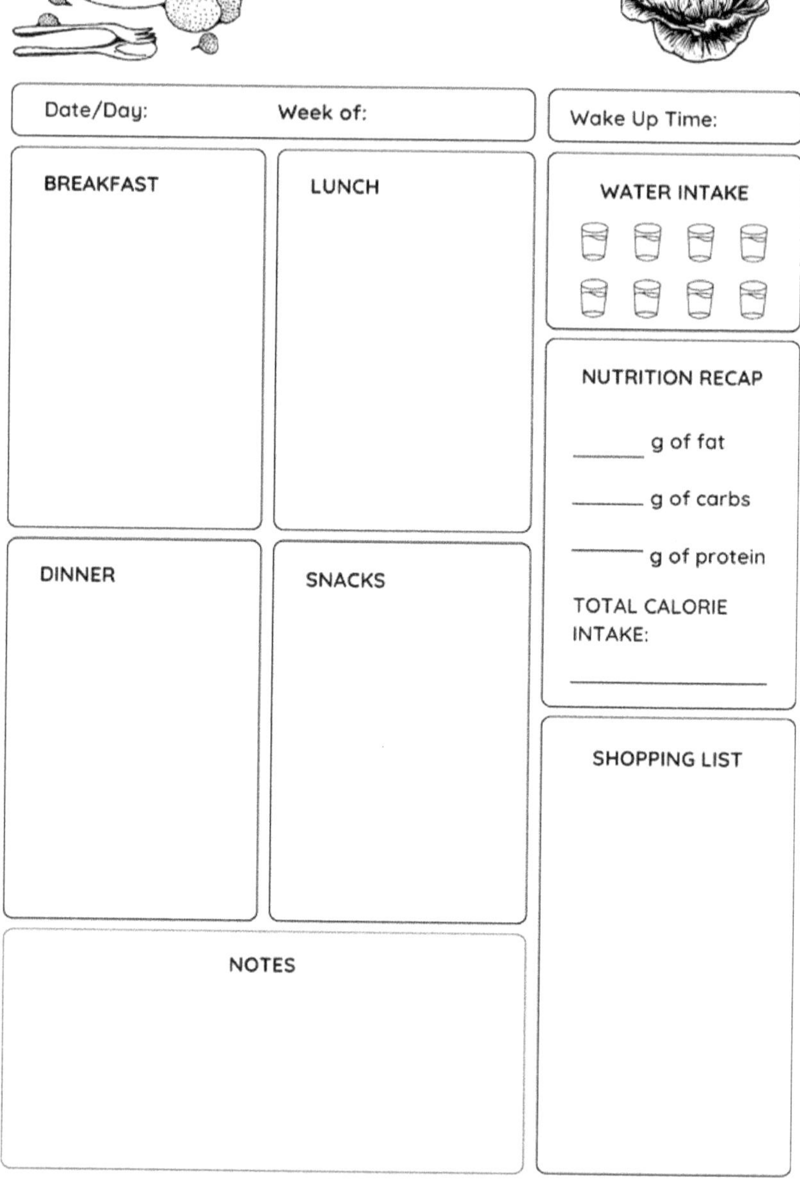
Date/Day:
Week of:
Wake Up Time:
BREAKFAST
LUNCH
WATER INTAKE
NUTRITION RECAP
_______ g of fat
_______ g of carbs
_______ g of protein
TOTAL CALORIE INTAKE:
DINNER
SNACKS
SHOPPING LIST
NOTES

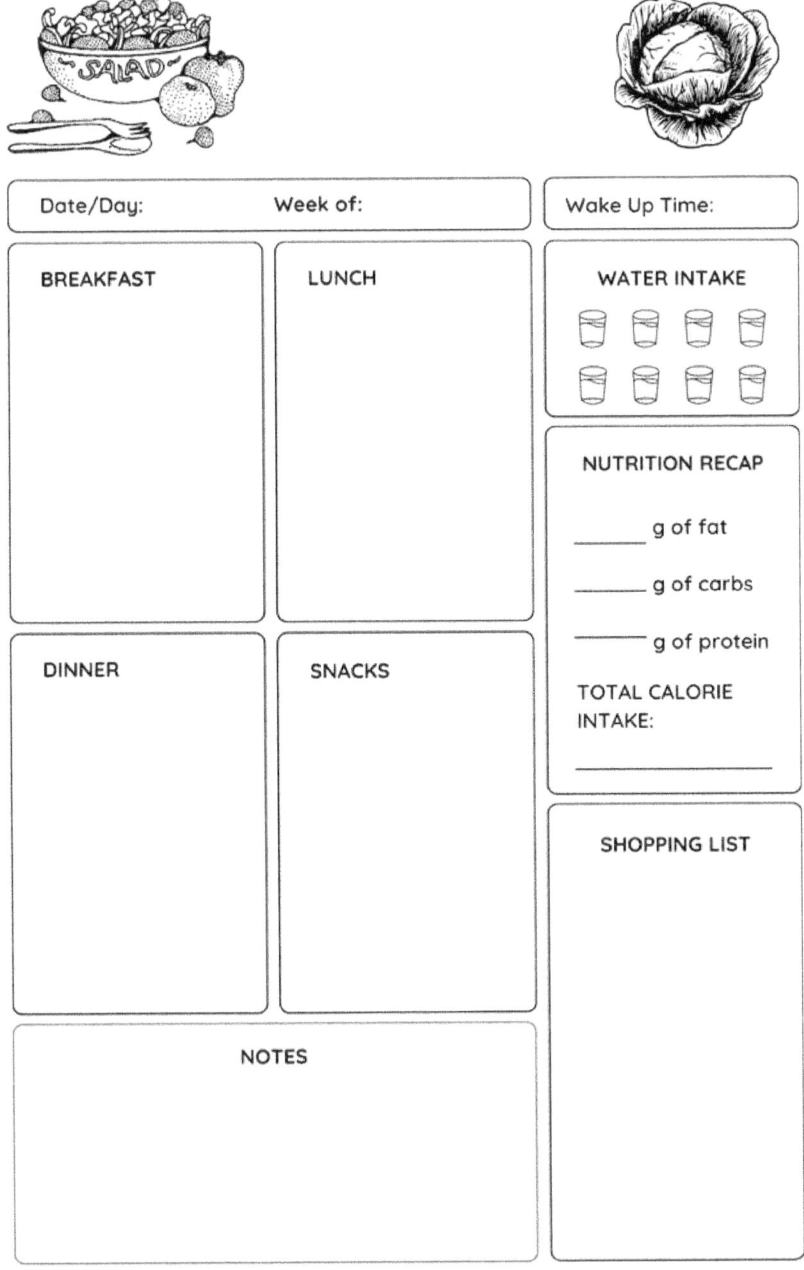

| Date/Day: | Week of: | Wake Up Time: |

**BREAKFAST**

**LUNCH**

**WATER INTAKE**

**NUTRITION RECAP**

_________ g of fat

_________ g of carbs

_________ g of protein

**TOTAL CALORIE INTAKE:**

____________________

**DINNER**

**SNACKS**

**SHOPPING LIST**

**NOTES**

www.ingramcontent.com/pod-product-compliance
Lightning Source LLC
Chambersburg PA
CBHW050817260726
48660CB00004B/1475